Beeson

PHYSICIAN PROFILING

Background and Practical Experience

Edited by
Kenneth J. Pechman, PhD, MD

American College of Physician Executives
Suite 200
4890 West Kennedy Boulevard
Tampa, Florida 33609
813/287-2000

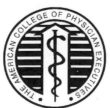

ISBN: 0-924674-74-1

Library of Congress Card Number: 99-067754

Printed in the United States of America by Hillsboro Printing Company, Tampa, Florida

CONTENTS

Preface i

Foreword iii

Acknowledgement v

SECTION I   The Rise of Physician Profiling

   Chapter 1   Practicing Medicine in America **3**
               Derick P. Pasternak, MD, MBA, FACPE

   Chapter 2   The Rise of Profiling **17**
               Marilyn Szymialis Radke, MD, MPH, MA, FACPM,
               CPE, FACPE

SECTION II   Issues and Concerns in Physician Profiling

   Chapter 3   Elements of a Physician Profile **37**
               Jonathan Bogen, MSPH, MBA, CHE

   Chapter 4   The Use and Misuse of Physician Profiles **51**
               Joseph A. Berry, MD, MBA

   Chapter 5   The Process of Physician Profiling **61**
               John R. Coombs, MD, and Margaret H.
               Gilshannon, MHA

   Chapter 6   The Legal Status of Provider Profiles **85**
               Todd Sagin, MD, JD

   Chapter 7   The Informatics of Physician Profiling **101**
               David M. Klubert, MD, and Colt G. Courtright, MPA

SECTION III   Physician Profiling in Practice

Chapter 8   Hospital Physician Profiling: Education-Based **135**
Practice Pattern Analysis
Frederic G. Jones, MD, CPE, FACPE, and
Craig C. Johnson, MHA, MPH

Chapter 9   A Medical Group Practice Looks Back on **149**
Physician Profiling...and Forward
Angelo P. Spoto, Jr. MD, FACP

Chapter 10   Physician Profiling in Managed Care
Orgainzations **161**
John M. Ludden, MD, CPE, FACPE

Chapter 11   Profiling at the Department of Veterans Affairs . . . **169**
James Arnold Tuchschmidt, MD, MBA, and
Carol M. Ashton, MD, MPH

Chapter 12   Profiling in an Academic Health Center **185**
Charles W. Mercer, MD, FACPE, John W.
Lacey, MD, and Francis Weisner, RN

Chapter 13   The Pharmacy Benefits Manager Perspective **189**
George Fulop, MD, MSCM, Glen Stettin, MD,
Wai Mo, Matt Donaldson

Index **201**

PREFACE

At the first meeting of the American College of Physician Executives' Forum on Quality Health Care Management in 1995, a group of about 20 physicians gathered to learn about profiling. Clearly most of the people attending the forum knew less than desired about profiling, but they expressed a definite interest in learning more. Some time after the meeting, discussions were held about drafting a book on the subject from the perspective of how profiling came about, what profiles were, and how people were applying the technique to the real world. Over the past 15 months, a number of contributors were sought and commissioned to explore the topic from different viewpoints. These viewpoints are assembled here to help the reader understand some of the issues surrounding physician profiling. The book is divided into three section, each addressing a different aspect of the profile management tool:

■ The rise of the physician profile.

■ Issues surrounding physician profiling.

■ Management applications of physician profiling.

The Rise of the Physician Profile

Since the turn of the century, the medical profession has been changing from a cottage industry to a business. The art of medicine has been altered by the science of medicine and its often lucrative and expensive technological advancements. As new treatments and devices were introduced to the armamentarium of the health care industry, valid questions were raised about the value of those treatments relative to their costs. The availability of financial resources, stretched to their limits, has become a barrier to further unbridled expansion. What is the value of the treatment or the diagnostic study to the patient, to the employer or third party payer, and to society? To control rising costs and to ensure value for the dollar of care purchased, one would naturally expect the introduction of management tools, continuing the conversion of the medical industry to a business. Section I looks at changes in the health care environment, changes in physician life-style expectations, and pressures that gave rise to the profiling of health care (and physicians).

Issues Surrounding Physician Profiling

A series of questions and concerns come to mind for those about to engage in the profiling process. The questions are not much different from those encountered by physicians engaging in the process or already under its scrutiny. A fair amount of distrust exists about the process. Will one be judged fairly against the experience of one's peers? What about severity of disease and patient mix in a physician's panel compared to those in the set of profiled physicians? Will the process profile health care or economic outcomes? After introducing the elements of a physician profile and exploring the process itself, this section explores some of the concerns about the use of profiling data in malpractice cases and in credentialing and about matters of confidentiality. Profiling is a data-intensive process. The adequacy of data collection, cross referencing of data sets, and various issues in data analysis conclude the section.

Management Applications of Physician Profiling

The final section of the book relates the profiling experience of several organizations and provides a basis of comparison of one's own organization to those included here. To provide a range of experiences, several types of organizations are represented, including a teaching hospital, a multispecialty medical group, a large medical health plan, a government organization, an academic center, and a pharmacy benefits plan. The range of types of organizations and how they are applying the tools of physician profiling should give the reader ample exposure to a wide range of experiences and an opportunity to network with those who may be facing similar experiences.

FOREWORD

Care providers desire to deliver the right care at the right time and in the right amount, each time and every time. Perhaps. In an ideal world, such would be the case, but the real world adds multifactorial variation, contributing to the differences seen in care giving. As the medical industry has moved from a patch quilt of interacting and sometimes conflicting parts to increasingly larger and more complex organizations, the opportunity to measure, and hence to manage, the quality of care has increased. Both growth of medical organizations and consolidation of the medical marketplace have fostered the application of management science to the complex medical care system. The cost of waste generated through variation of care had been hidden in cost-plus operations in previous decades. Rising costs and managed care growth have forced optimization rather than maximization in health care delivery.

The introduction of management of care has not always come easily. Physicians have studied long hours and trained hard to deliver what they individually felt was the best care for the situations at hand. They have come to expect to be compensated for their efforts on the basis of the complexity of that process and the technological status of procedures or treatments and, perhaps, because they and not an alternative care provider or physician extender have rendered the care. As management of the health care profession advances, payment for outcomes rather than for process will require a change in the mindset of physicians and their practice managers. It will be important to know if one is a cost-effective provider, not only relative to one's peers but also relative to standards accepted in the industry. As medical informatics applications become more widespread and more sophisticated, the ability to effectively hide behind the numbers will be reduced.

Profiling is now and will continue to be a tool used widely in the profession and on the profession by outsiders. Insurers, employers, and patients will be able to access more and more information about their doctors and hospitals and about health care issues pertinent to them. The medical profession should address the use of profiling and other management tools in a proactive manner to gain the information needed to improve their care delivery and to be able to prove that improved care is delivered to those who would ask.

Recently, 186 physicians, ranging from CEOs to medical directors participated in a CyberForum on physician profiling sponsored by the American College of Physician Executives. The CyberForum discussions demonstrate that there is a wide range of applications and sophistication in applications of the profiling process in the industry. The one constant across the field was the need to improve the process where it was already in place and to engage in the process where it was not. Participants raised a number of issues during the forum and sought practical experience in profiling from their colleagues.

The rise of the physician profile is explored in the Physician Profiling: Background and Practical Experience. The book serves as a guide through a number of issues and concerns, including informatics, legal risk, uses and abuses of the process, and others. How are organizations employing the tool? Several examples are presented to provide some insight into applications of profiling. Profiling should be embraced as a tool to benefit both the provider and the recipient of care and not viewed as a punishment or a burden to the provider. As Dr. Radke states in chapter 2, "The ultimate goal of profiling is to improve health care by making medical practice more appropriate and cost-effective."

ACKNOWLEDGMENT

This book would not exist without the efforts of many people. First, the many authors who unselfishly contributed their respective chapters are thanked for their insight and cooperation. Appreciation for their support and understanding are due to my staff, Nancy, Holly, Sparky, and Kathy. To my family, thank you for your patience and continued understanding throughout the process. And finally, a big thank you to Wes Curry, whose gentle guidance and insight were instrumental in bringing this project to fruition.

SECTION I

The Rise of Physician Profiling

CHAPTER 1

*Practicing Medicine
in America*
by Derick P. Pasternak, MD, MBA, FACPE

*I*n the early 1980s, when Paul Starr's major study of U.S. medical practice was published, few chose to dispute this assessment of the profession: "In America no one group has held so dominant a position in this new world of rationality and power as has the medical profession."[1] Physicians enjoyed unprecedented social status and prosperity all through the 1970s, due at least in part to their ability to turn expanding government and private health insurance coverage into economic advantage. Moreover, the rapid advancement of diagnostic and therapeutic technologies, fueled in part by hospitals' willingness to invest in any new technology in the era of cost-based reimbursement and capital pass-throughs, created a widening range of physician earning power at the top end. Although society was beginning to protest the high price of health care, few, if any, observers predicted the drastic changes that were in store for insurers, doctors, hospitals, and patients alike.

Young physicians entering the profession at the turn of the 21st Century have a vastly different professional life to anticipate from their colleagues who completed their medical education in the 1970s and earlier. Almost every aspect of patient care has changed in the past thirty years, some slightly, some drastically. Through the first two thirds of the century, most physicians practiced in solo or small group settings, beholden to practically no one except for a need to be affable enough to maintain a word-of-mouth reputation. Most physicians, other than surgeons who removed tissue at operations, were able to keep the results of their ministrations to themselves—if they bothered to keep track of them at all. The noncompetitive, "there is enough for everyone" status of medicine fostered collegiality and affability among practitioners, which at the same time inhibited honest feedback when such was needed, except for infrequent cases.

The medical profession was able to perform in this unstructured manner because society presumed that the United States had the highest quality of medical care anywhere on Earth, and individual physicians were all presumed to have been equally well trained. The hard work physicians-in-training were known to have been subjected to was assumed to have ensured that everyone who got through it was a high-quality practitioner. Physicians' professional opinions were seldom challenged and were almost never required to be backed by evidence, except in the rare academic settings.

The Employed Physician

By the 1970s, physicians were congregating in group practices in steadily increasing numbers. The institutions established between 1890 and the 1920s (Mayo, Geisinger, Henry Ford, Cleveland, and others) grew steadily, surpassing every prediction of optimal size for a medical group, at which they were supposed to stop growing. Younger groups followed suit, in at least one instance (Permanente Medical Group) already matching the size of the giants. Since then, there has been rapid consolidation, with groups becoming institutions, diversifying geographically as well as professionally. A sign of the times was the decision in 1992 by the American Group Practice Association (now named the American Medical Group Association) to proclaim itself the voice of large vertically integrated multispecialty group practices, even when the majority of its member groups had fewer than 100 physicians.[2]

Today, the typical physician completing postgraduate training is more likely than ever before to seek long-term employment with an institution that may offer various practice sites and a variety of practice styles. Alternatively, young physicians may enter government employment, because state and federal governments have become direct providers of health care. Whether the group is government employment, equity-model, foundation-model, or staff-model, physicians enter a setting that makes them feel like employees, not decision makers (owners or managers). Physician practice management companies, particularly if publicly traded, also provide an ambiance of working for someone else.[3] The employee mind-set of young physicians has profound consequences on the way they practice their profession. Work rules are promulgated, often without input by physicians; patient flow and appointment schedules are controlled by persons other than the practitioner; and formularies, disease management protocols, hospital admission and discharge criteria and record-keeping requirements appear, as if from nowhere, to constrain what had in the past been an almost unfettered ability of the physician to make professional decisions.

Unlike the private or small group practice setting, the institutional setting discourages physicians from mixing their professional and private lives. Someone may keep an eye on time off, on private long distance telephone calls, or on use of e-mail for private purposes. This type of intrusiveness, taken for granted in practically every industry, is a new experience for physicians, especially for those who did not enter the institutional setting directly from training. Although data in this area are scarce, it is the author's belief that insurance company-owned and hospital-sponsored institutions, even when proclaimed to be "physician-driven," have more in common with government employment models than with historically physician-dominated group practices. Keeping private life out of the workplace is often coupled by a feature found to be desirable by young physicians: keeping the workplace out of the home. On call schedules are sharply circumscribed, and, as far as possible, minimized; telephone hot-lines and other devices are used to reduce after-hours obligations of doctors to their patients. Inpatient specialists with well-defined work schedules are often available to reduce or eliminate hospital obligations of physicians.

The changes just described, coupled with significant changes in professional practice, create an industrialized setting of medicine, leaving behind the cottage-industry features that characterized it until recently. Not too surprisingly, another aspect of industrial employment has appeared among physician-employees as well: labor union membership. Aside from the 20,000 or more physicians-in-training who have been able to join unions in some instances since the 1960s,[4] physicians have begun to turn to unions as their collective bargaining agents in government and private for-profit and not-for-profit settings.[5,6]

Changes in Professional Practice

Among the most cherished traditions of medical practitioners has been professional autonomy. The wide diversity of patients, and of the way in which they present themselves when ill, has served as a reason (excuse) for many physicians to refuse to acknowledge the need for standard approaches to most common illnesses. Even surgical specialists, who were trained to adopt standard operative procedures, referred to "surgical judgment" as an overriding consideration when they were discovered not to have followed standards.

At its best, the diversity of approaches allowed physicians to make special allowances for variation in patient anatomy and physiology, for coexisting or complicating conditions, or for idiosyncratic or otherwise unexpected patient responses to treatments administered. All too often, however, "physician judgment" was used to avoid accountability for the outcomes of care. Even in settings in which review of practices was routinely done (surgical case reviews, morbidity and mortality conferences, etc.), it was the exception, rather than the rule, to subject a colleague to the kind of scrutiny that was implied by the high-minded phrase, "peer review."

The almost continuous malpractice crises of the 1970s and 1980s succeeded in penetrating the veil of "physician judgment." First, a common standard within a specialty was articulated and eventually adopted as a medicolegal principle, even while general practitioners were held to the looser "community standard." Later, as general practitioners were increasingly replaced by board-certified family practitioners, general internists, and internist/pediatricians, the latter were subjected by the courts to the same national specialty standard as other specialists. However, in most instances, the courts accepted the testimony of a suitably credentialed expert as to standards[7]; in case of conflicting expert testimony, the jury was allowed to define the standard from among the alternatives presented. This was both a cumbersome and an inconsistent approach. It is not surprising that this definition did not lead to widespread acceptance among physicians, other than recognition in professional circles that some standards may be desirable. By coming to terms with the notion, if not the specific application, of professional standards, physicians began to edge closer to accepting accountability in a systematic fashion, rather than just by the hit or miss method of being called to account in a civil lawsuit.

The growth of group practices also favored physicians' acceptance of standards of practice. By the mid 1980s, more than 30 percent of physicians were practicing in groups through a variety of employment models, a proportion that has increased since then. There were several ways in which groups fostered accountability:

- Sharing practices increased the frequency of informal consultations and communications about patient care issues. Physicians became familiar with one another's practice styles, perhaps idiosyncrasies. This led not only to accommodation but also, through a subtle process, to a gradual convergence of styles.

- The convergence of styles became more pronounced through regular sharing of on-call duties. Among the benefits of group practice perceived by physicians was the limitation of on-call hours and the increase in paid time off (even if productivity-based compensation discouraged taking the time off in many instances).

- Larger and more established groups, especially those with academic ties, began to formalize the standard-setting process by duplicating the peer review functions originally established in hospitals as part of the quality measurement and management function, driven mostly by JCAHO requirements.

- As groups became providers of health care under managed care arrangements, quality reviews and accountability became more prevalent.[8]

In 1966, the federal government became the most prominent source of financing of health care services through Medicare, and subsequently through other programs that financed care delivered through the private sector. (We will not consider the Veterans' Administration, Uniformed Services, and Federal Bureau of Prisons here—if anything, the health care delivered in these settings changed after the changes occurred in the private sector.) For about 10 years, the Medicare program caused little change in the way physicians provided care; the rapid growth of costs, however, caused extensive investigation into physician practices, which is ongoing today, more than three decades after passage of the legislation. Through utilization review, mandatory in hospitals and duplicated at the professional standards review organization (PSRO) and then the peer review organization (PRO) level, practices that wasted government funds without benefit or with questionable benefit to patients were supposed to be eliminated. At the same time, quality assurance was established for the purpose implicit in the name of the function. The reception of these efforts in the medical community can only be described as hostile. Physicians were unused to the notion that the party that paid the bills had any right to review the content or the outcomes of care. The author recalls an incident from the late 1970s during which a PSRO quality assurance committee indicated to a group of doctors that their record of only 30 percent positive pathology following primary, nonincidental appendectomy may not reflect optimal care. The helpful reply from the physicians in question suggested producing several copies of the letter, chopping them up finely, and using the product to blanket the countryside in order to ensure a good crop that year!

With the advent of the Medicare prospective payment system in the early 1980s, the government's approach changed. The system now provided incentives to hospitals for reducing the resources devoted to every Medicare patient admitted. PROs were now to abandon looking at possible overutilization, and to look instead for evidence of needed treatment being withheld. This focus highlighted the almost total lack of authoritative guidelines for treatment of most common conditions. As the federal government began to look for ways to remedy this situation, it set in motion (or accelerated) forces that brought about a drastic transformation in the way in which physicians approach patient care. This transformation is a long way from being complete at this time, but it has gathered momentum.

The change is by no means an easy one. Gone are the jocose responses that compare government or managed care mandates to fertilizer; replaced by invective, political pressure, and lawsuits to force provision of services, even some that are of questionable benefit. Nonetheless, the change is inexorable; whenever a physician interacts with a patient today, there are three sets of influences on the choice of therapies that will be delivered or recommended:

- The patient's complaint, or diagnosis, if known, and coexisting conditions.

- The economics of the care setting.

- Guidelines and other professional support structure available for delivering care for patients with the given presenting problem.

Effects of Changes in Financing Health Care

In addition to changes in Medicare policies, the increased prevalence of managed care, with its heavy emphasis on intrusive review of physicians' practices, caused drastic changes in the way in which physicians conduct their office practices.

In the mid 1970s, it was still believed that the changes in health care financing that were prevalent in California and other West Coast locations would not spread to the rest of the country. It was widely presumed that Americans would not accept the kind of constraints that closed-panel HMOs such as Kaiser, Group Health Cooperative of Puget Sound, or the Ross-Loos Clinic represented. To be sure, a few communities experimented with small managed care plans, while representing to physicians that their practice style would not have to change. However, when it became clear that the latter assurance was wishful thinking at best, fraudulent misrepresentation at worst, there was an expectation that prepaid plans in each market would remain small, with insignificant penetration of the market, much as Health Insurance Plan of New York existed for decades without being able to expand its model.

The inexorable rise in health care costs, however, aroused employers, who eventually concluded that inconveniencing employees was preferable to facing ever-increasing health care premiums. They found the means by which employees themselves made the choice of restricted networks in order to minimize their contributions to the premium paid. As a result, the managed care movement expanded, slowly in some places, more rapidly elsewhere. From Alabama to Washington, from Nevada to New Hampshire, managed care contracting has become a skill as necessary for physicians as taking a history or delivering an infant. Those who did not understand that fact or who chose to "tough it out" suffered severe economic consequences; others either joined an institutional practice or, together with colleagues, created infrastructures such as individual practice associations (IPAs).

In addition to dealing with contracting complexities presented by managed care, physicians had to provide access to their medical records for a number of economic and clinical auditing activities. Specialist referrals, hospitalizations, certain radiologic procedures and other tests, and durable medical equipment all became subject to a prior approval process. Finally, with increasing frequency, physicians had to demonstrate that they complied with certain clinical guidelines and the recommendations embodied in the standards known as HEDIS (Health Plan Data and Information Set).[9]

Practice Guidelines

The Agency for Health Care Policy and Research (AHCPR) represents a government effort to develop industrywide standards in health care. With these standards, the task of evaluating the appropriateness of services performed and the effectiveness in the way they are performed becomes easier. Throughout its brief existence, AHCPR has been under pressure because its own performance was initially questionable and because the political process has been used by many to resist the trends that the agency represented. Nonetheless, the agency has now survived long enough to have several accomplishments to its credit, among which has been the publication of practice guidelines for conditions as wide ranging as congestive heart failure, low back pain, and breast cancer, among others.[10] Political pressures compelled AHCPR to stop issuing new guidelines in 1996, but the extant ones have been widely used as benchmarks.

Practice guidelines have been the subject of activity in three other types of organizations: the physician-driven multispecialty groups already mentioned, especially those with heavy or exclusive managed care activity (e.g., the staff-model Harvard Community Health Plan in the early 1980s); physician professional societies (including, as of 1997, the American Medical Association), and academic and research settings. The focus of the first type of organization was internal use. Their motivation was similar to the government's: develop a set of algorithms that will enable the organization to distinguish between appropriate and inappropriate services and that will facilitate measurement of quality of care. For organizations that were at economic risk because they assumed global capitation, this was an endeavor that served an economic purpose as well and was worth the investment in time and manpower. Professional societies, on the other hand, may have had different and probably more complex motivation for this activity, because they had no economic risk. They represent groups of physicians, however, who were faced with government's or their own administrators' (even if physician administrators) presuming to prescribe how to care for patients they frequently treated. Whatever the reasons, many societies published guidelines of their own. At times, this resulted in different societies' publishing guidelines that were in conflict with one another. The most prominent of these conflicts was the guideline for performing screening mammography, which became a political as well as a professional controversy. Finally, independent research organizations and academic institutions have been active in the development of guidelines[11] as they sought ways in which their research could be more relevant to changing health care.

Practice guidelines were being developed parallel to the implementation of continuous quality improvement (CQI) in health care organizations. Conceptually, the two approaches were compatible, because CQI in any industry requires that processes be defined prior to being improved, and guidelines define medical processes, frequently for the first time. Despite this congruence, in many settings the initiatives were not seen as two parts of a whole, but rather as two disconnected and confusing efforts, both aimed at reducing physician autonomy. Many physicians were unconvinced that care would really improve as a result of all of this; they presumed that all efforts were designed to control costs.[12] Because multispecialty groups and managed care plans represented a minority of care settings, most medical practitioners were able to remain unaffected by guidelines and CQI through the 1980s and early 1990s.

One effort to broaden the use of guidelines was the action of a state to accept evidence of a physician's following a published guideline as defense in malpractice action. Because of the proliferation of conflicting guidelines, or for other reasons, this approach did not become widely adopted.

Disease Management

Recognition among leaders of medical institutions that CQI, guidelines, and other activities aimed at ensuring high-quality care were getting indifferent reactions from most physicians led to the disease management movement. Disease management, as we understand it today, focuses all the tools of quality assessment and improvement into concrete clinical settings. Most disease management activities revolve around frequently treated conditions (e.g., congestive heart failure in the elderly, asthma in children) or around conditions that, while not major public health problems, nonetheless affect the patient population significantly and are subjects of society's special interest (e.g., depression, breast cancer). The interest of certain pharmaceutical companies in the disease management approach also resulted in less common conditions' being the subject of projects establishing disease management protocols (epilepsy, peptic ulcer disease). Whatever the source of these projects, their clinical orientation and practical approach has awakened physician interest.[13]

Disease management is the embodiment of population-based medical care. When a health care institution assumes responsibility for care of a defined population, the institution and its professionals must approach the care of individual patients in a manner that will preserve resources in order to provide optimal care and services to the entire population, not just the person across the desk, on the examining table, or in a hospital bed. In order to perform optimally, physicians and other members of the healthcare team must pay special attention to those conditions that consume a large proportion of the resources available for the whole population. Disease management identifies major processes that make up the totality of care for a certain condition (e.g. asthma). Then, through the Deming-Shewhart cycle, the processes are defined and improved. Finally, through the disease management process, outcomes of the entire episode, not just the individual care components, are measured and reported.

Physicians play major roles in disease management. They are on design teams, on which they invariably assume leadership position, and they are the major, although not exclusive, agents carrying out the processes that make up the disease management approach to patient care. By virtue of the license they possess, they have nearly exclusive right to prescribe medications (e.g., inhaled steroids for asthma) or to perform surgical procedures (e.g., tracheostomy). In most situations, they decide what resources will be used in the treatment of individual patients (e.g., pulmonary function tests, allergy tests, inpatient treatment). In our society, they also take the responsibility when things go wrong (e.g., being sued for malpractice). Because of the sharp clinical focus of disease management, it has been an approach that has enlisted support from many physicians, generalists and specialists alike.

Although all physicians are exposed to the principles of population-based medicine through public health courses during their training, this exposure has for most been of little relevance to their professional careers. Population-based medicine and disease management apply the principles of public health in the day-to-day practice of physicians. At the same time, the physician is comfortable with his or her role as patient advocate, because the outcome monitoring piece of disease management ensures that economics are not the only goal.

The process we call "disease management" has been implemented in a multiplicity of ways. Sometimes, the appellation is merely applied to a few protocols; sometimes, extensive new structures, such as disease- or treatment-specific clinics, are organized. In a number of well-organized institutions, literally dozens of disease management protocols, complete with process improvement teams, clinical and economic outcome measurement, and research and development of further protocols and programs have become part of the management of professional practice.

Primary Care Practice

The primary care practitioner today is charged with maintaining the time-tested role of being his patients' main health care advisor and most frequently used caregiver, while also carrying out the following functions:

■ Keeping track of health care financing of each patient in order to be certain that all referral and utilization rules are observed.

■ Influencing acute care hospital utilization of his or her panel of managed care patients.

■ Performing or keeping track of preventive services provided to his or her panel of managed care patients.

■ Keeping track of diverse and changing specialist panels maintained by the various managed care plans.

■ Keeping track of pharmaceutical costs and using various formularies as required by managed care plans.

■ Communicating with specialists.

■ Selectively referring to specialists within the panels who have demonstrated cost-effective practices as well as clinical excellence.

■ Training and overseeing an office staff that will collect and update demographic information, record diagnoses and procedures correctly, generate correct bills and send them out on time, and keep track of accounts receivable.

All of these functions have to be performed in an environment that is also characterized by laws that restrict the ability of the physician to gain from certain practices, by tightening regulatory oversight by government at all levels, by more intense competition from nonphysician providers of care, and by a need for more continuing medical education in order to maintain relicensure and recertification.

Although these requirements are imposed on primary care physicians, there are resources that help them meet them. Many of these resources are electronically based information systems. They carry both an economic cost and the need for physicians to become computer literate.

Specialty Care Practice

Today's specialists operate on the horns of a dilemma. On the one hand, managed care and government-financed care create an imperative to perform or order only services that can be justified through reference to standard guidelines; criteria; or, in the case of Medicare and Medicaid, federal and state regulation. On the other hand, improved diagnostic and therapeutic capabilities, as well as expectations of well-informed patients, create enthusiasm for use of new modalities (e.g., surgical procedures) before they have been conclusively proven beneficial. Specialists, more than primary care physicians, dread the specter of medical malpractice lawsuits if all possible treatments are not administered to a given patient and the patient does not have a good outcome.

In addition to the above, specialists have a multiplicity of networks and managed care plans to keep track of, frequently with very different financing mechanisms. All specialists also have to contend with the following functions (which are similar to those above for primary care physicians):

■ Keeping track of pharmaceutical costs and using various formularies as required by managed care plans.

■ Communicating with primary care physicians.

■ Selectively referring to colleagues within the panels who have demonstrated cost-effective practices as well as clinical excellence. (This is especially true for specialists who are subcapitated or are paid through so-called carve-out arrangements.)

■ Training and overseeing an office staff that will collect and update demographic information, record diagnoses and procedures correctly, generate correct bills and send them out on time, and keep track of accounts receivable.

Finally, the environmental constraints already mentioned, such as licensure, recertification, federal and state laws, and regulations relating relationships to hospitals are major concerns. In addition, some specialists, such as ophthalmologists, orthopedists, obstetricians, and anesthesiologists, are pressured by competition from nonphysicians who seek to provide care to the same group of patients.

Physician Profiling as an Aid to Medical Practice

Whereas physician profiling is not used for the primary purpose of aiding the individual physician in his or her daily practice, many organizations that conduct profiling have used the process in a way that enables them to use published profiles as tools to help themselves and their patients. Profiling has evolved from a strictly score-keeping tool for use by insurance company medical directors to become the subject of meaningful feedback to caregivers. Today's physician profiles are often presented in easy to interpret graphic formats with backup by encounter-based data. Interpretation of the graphs, as well as documentation of changing practice over time, is sometimes included in the communication. Profiles remain out of phase, however. They frequently report events that occurred 6 to 24 months earlier. Because practice patterns may have changed drastically in the interim (new drugs being released, new surgical procedures utilized), this timing problem limits the usefulness of profiles to the practicing doctor.

Factual, rather than normative presentation of data that can be shown to be accurate is likely to elicit at least curiosity from physicians who are subjects of profiling. At best, physicians react to the data by changing their behavior to conform with what they perceive as best practices. This will always include physicians who have been documented to yield the best clinical outcomes. If the physician's economic incentives are properly aligned, his or her definition of best practice will also extend to the cost-effectiveness aspect of the outcome.

Not all physicians will respond spontaneously to their practice profiles. Sometimes the lack of response is caused by a lack of understanding of the relevance of the data. At other times, physicians will be unable to adopt an alternate approach to certain patients because of ingrained habits or a lack of exposure to new or at least different ways of approaching disease entities or patient complaints. Even in this situation, however, profiles communicated in a non-adversarial fashion and unaccompanied by mandates or other means of compulsion function as supportive background for further customized intervention by a managed care medical director or another appropriate change agent.

Physicians in group practices (equity or employment model) are in the best position to use profiling as a tool to improve the cost-effectiveness and the outcome of the care provided. They have mechanisms already established through which all relevant data, including profiles, can be reviewed and analyzed and action can be taken for improvement. As already mentioned, most group practice physicians are already accustomed to reviewing and influencing one anothers' work. Physician profiles become simply another type of input that they use in their work life. As profiling becomes more sophisticated and real-time, it no doubt will have even greater influence on the ability of physicians to respond rapidly to the need to change in order to be successful, professionally and economically.

References

1. Starr, P. *The Social Transformation of American Medicine.* New York, N.Y.: Basic Books, 1982. p. 4.

2. AGPA Board of Trustees. *AGPA-2000: A Vision. A Long Range and Strategic Action Plan.* Alexandria, Va.: American Group Practice Association, 1992.

3. Pasternak, D. "Practice Management Companies: What Do They Offer Physicians?" *Frontiers of Health Services Management* 14(2):47-51, Winter 1997.

4. Moran, M. "Residents Regret Signing on with Union, Seek to Disaffiliate." *American Medical News* 1998; 41(3):6, Jan. 19, 1998.

5. Azevedo, D. "Taking Back Health Care: New Owners Drive This Group to Unionize." *Medical Economics* 74(6):194-207, March 24, 1997.

6. Jaklevic, M. "Trying to Be Heard. Docs Employed by Hospitals, Systems Seek to Unionize." *Modern Healthcare* 28(14):32, April 6, 1998.

7. "Selected Recent Court Cases; Blood Industry Standard of Care." *American Journal of Law and Medicine* 18(3):281-2, Summer 1992.

8. Luft, H. "Modifying Managed Competition to Address Cost and Quality." *Health Affairs* 15(1):23-38, Spring 1996.

9. NCQA Reference Set. *Book III, HEDIS 3.0/1998.* Washington, D.C.: National Committee for Quality Assurance, 1997.

10. For instance, AHCPR Panel, A*cute Low Back Problems in Adults, Clinical Practice Guideline Number 14.* Rockville, Md.: U.S. Department of Health and Human Service, Public Health Service, Agency for Health Care Policy and Research, 1994. AHCPR Panel, *Post-Stroke Rehabilitation: Assessment, Referral, and Patient Management, Quick Reference Guide for Clinicians Number 16.* Rockville, Md.: U.S. Department of Health and Human Service, Public Health Service, Agency for Health Care Policy and Research, 1995.

11. Frances, A., and others. "A New Method of Developing Expert Consensus Practice Guidelines." *American Journal of Managed Care* 4(7):1023-9, July 1998.

12. Pasternak, D., and Lucas, J. "Culture Change: Clinical Practice Improvement at Lovelace Health Systems." *Group Practice Journal* 43(4):26-31, July-Aug. 1994.

13. Harris, J. "Disease Management; New Wine in New Bottles?" *Annals of Internal Medicine* 124(9):838-42, May 1, 1996.

Derick P. Pasternak, MD, MBA, FACPE, is Chief Executive, Providence Puget Sound Service Area, Seattle, Washington.

CHAPTER 2

The Rise of Profiling

Marilyn Szymialis Radke, MD, MPH, MA, FACPM, CPE, FACPE

*P*hysician profiling is a natural reaction to changes in the environment as medicine has been transformed from a cottage industry to big business. Marketplace pressures demand efficient and effective medical care. To survive in this competitive environment, physicians must balance access to their services with efficient practice patterns.[1] Practice guidelines, medical effectiveness and outcomes research, and quality management techniques designed to identify problems and improve performance are evolving to address the challenges of the American health care system concerning cost and quality. Profiling has emerged as an important tool in these diverse efforts to understand medical care production by comparing physician practice patterns. Profiling has an impact on medical practice and can play a role in quality improvement, assessment of provider performance, and utilization review and in improving health care delivery in general.[2]

Corporate medicine holds physicians accountable and assesses their professional performance. Every professional is subject to profiling when society has the technology and economic incentive to perform profiling. Attorneys' performance is measured by the number of articles they publish in legal journals, the proportion of cases they win for their clients, the income and clients they bring to their law firms, and the profits (or losses) of their firms. The performance of management consultants and accountants is measured in a similar way. Professionals in many occupations are profiled by the key outcomes of the persons producing them. The better the outcome, the more valuable is the person producing it. In the marketplace, the customer wants and pays for outcomes, not for the processes used or the education, training, experience, or hard work that goes into producing those outcomes. Competition and commerce depend on the standardized measurement of these outcomes, i.e., goods and services produced and traded.[3]

Most performance assessment focuses on lengths of stay, readmissions, and other data that indicate how physicians and groups practice procedurally. The connection to patient outcomes, patient satisfaction, and functional status is missing, because outcome measures are lacking. Performance assessment criteria used by managed care to profile physicians and groups include utilization measures (inpatient days per thousand patients, referrals to specialists, ancillary tests, and emergency department visits), cost measures (monthly cost per member), and quality measures (member satisfaction surveys, transfer and termination rates, adherence to practice guidelines, and chart audits).[4]

Medicine is a competitive business in which contracts between purchasers of care (employees and insurers) and providers (health care delivery systems) determine which providers treat which patients. As cost and quality considerations begin to blend, competition is increasingly based on the value of medical care. Physician performance assessment and profiling are evolving beyond being used almost exclusively as economic indicators.[4] Measuring processes of medicine helps to codify them into practice guidelines, and measuring outcomes helps to define the performance and to determine the market value of providers and health plans. The ability to measure and standardize processes and outcomes of medical care is increasing. For example, there are standardized nomenclatures for diagnoses and procedures (CPT-4 and ICD9-CM) and for patients' functional status (Short Form-36). Premium price and outcomes can differentiate health plans among purchasers and providers.[3] When used properly, profiling can encourage improvement in the quality of health care and control costs.[5]

The rationale for physician profiling arises from the finding that variation in physician behavior may or may not improve quality of care and may provide an opportunity for cost savings. Practice variation and standardization are related to many aspects of medical quality management, and physician profiling is a tool for utilization review and quality assurance.[5]

The Beginnings of Profiling

Although Codman proposed comparative performance measures for hospitals in 1916, the era of profiling in medicine began with hospitals in the 1980s. The Health Care Financing Administration (HCFA) began the task for health care institutions nationally in 1987 when it paid hospitals fixed case rates for Medicare patients.[6] Hospitals then began to study the practice patterns of physicians whose orders for Medicare inpatient services determined whether or not hospitals made a profit on the care they delivered. At that time, most profiling was not shared with the physicians profiled.[3]

Physician profiling began with studies of variation in the use of surgical procedures such as transurethral resection of the prostate, cesarean sections, and ton-
sillectomies. These studies found a high degree of variation in physician use of
those procedures. Researchers seeking a cause for this variation found very little difference in population health and in the belief structures of physicians.
They found greater variation in the actual behavior of physicians. Analysis of
the quality and cost of health care among groups of physicians found that, if
there is no difference in quality between high-priced and low-priced groups,
there may be opportunity for cost savings. Variation did not add quality to
health care, but it did add cost.[5]

Release of physician-specific mortality rates for cardiac bypass surgery patients
in New York in 1991 was controversial.[6] The Physician Payment Review
Commission (PPRC) held a conference on practice pattern profiling in January
1992 and noted that patterns and organization of medical practice varied widely across the country and that there was uncertainty as to what approaches
worked best and how health care can be provided most efficiently. New diagnostic and treatment methods are increasingly complex and expensive. Some
patients may receive health care that is of little or no benefit to them, while others do not receive care that is known to be effective.[2] A wide range of institutions conduct provider profiling for a variety of purposes, including quality
improvement through provider feedback and education, provider selection and
credentialing, provider compensation, focused utilization review, provider marketing, and sanctions.[6]

States began collecting standardized outcomes measures of inpatients in the
1980s, and most states now collect a limited, standardized data set on inpatients, such as the uniform billing abstract (UB-92), which includes several
diagnosis and procedure codes. States also collect data on outpatient visits
for claims data from their Medicaid populations. Profiling of physicians'
practice patterns over episodes of illness are limited to insurers with large
claims databases. Insurers can use the profiles to select physicians and group
practices for their provider networks. Hospitals can use discharge data to
profile physicians' practice patterns for economic credentialing and can
withhold admitting privileges when practice patterns adversely affect the
economic performance of the hospital.[3]

The Methods of Profiling

Profiling is an analytic tool to assess health care delivery by focusing on patterns of care rather than on individual occurrences of care. Large databases
provide information to identify a health care provider's pattern of practice and
to compare it with patterns of similar providers or with accepted standards of
care. Profiling can identify over- and underutilization of services, problems

with the efficiency and quality of care, and provider performance issues. Profiling has broad applications for health care professionals, patients, payers, medical educators, and policy makers.[2]

Profiling uses epidemiological methods to compare practice patterns of health care providers regarding cost, service utilization, and quality (process and outcome) of health care. Providers, including individual practitioners, groups of practitioners, and health care organizations such as hospitals and managed care organizations, can be profiled. The provider's practice pattern is expressed as a profiling rate—a measure of utilization (costs or services) or outcome (functional status, morbidity, or mortality) aggregated over time for a defined population of patients under the provider's care during that time. For example, the number of sigmoidoscopy claims a physician submits to the Medicare program per 100 Medicare patients the physician sees in a given year is a utilization profiling rate.[2]

The utilization or outcome profiling rate for a particular provider is compared to a norm. A practice-based norm is a rate derived from the practice patterns of other similar providers. A standards-based norm is a rate that would be expected if providers followed an accepted practice guideline. Practice-based norms may or may not reflect appropriate care. Standards-based norms reflect appropriate care to the extent that accepted practice guidelines are based on scientific evidence.[2]

Profiles usually generate some type of action if utilization or the outcome profiling rate for a particular provider differs from the norm by a certain amount. For example, the Medicare program may notify an internist that his or her Medicare sigmoidoscopy rate is greater than two standard deviations above the mean for other internists practicing in the same community. The Medicare program may notify all internists how their Medicare sigmoidoscopy rates compare with a standards-based norm.[2]

By focusing on aggregate patterns rather than on patterns of individual practitioners, profiling can be used to compare the patterns of care provided by health care organizations or received by groups of patients. For example, profiling rates for outpatient sigmoidoscopy can be compared among different geographic regions of the country, profiling rates for cesarean section can be compared among managed care organizations, or profiling rates for mortality following coronary artery bypass surgery can be compared among hospitals.[2]

Profiling rates can be applied in quality improvement, assessment of provider performance, and utilization review. Quality improvement is the process of identifying and solving problems through changes in performance. Poor or variable outcomes often indicate problems in health care. Improving health care outcomes may depend on changes made by physicians, nonphysician practitioners, patients, or health care systems.[2]

Profiling may play a role in several aspects of quality improvement. It can identify conditions or procedures for which there are large variations in outcome. Profiling rates can target differences in specific outcome frequencies when patients with a particular condition or patients undergoing a particular procedure receive health care services from different providers.[2]

Profiling can help to determine how to change performance to improve outcome. Physicians may use outcome profile rates to identify specific differences in health care processes associated with differences in outcome. Quality improvement can result from profiling both process and outcome, seeking correlations between them, or changing a process across providers and re-profiling to assess whether differences in outcome decrease or overall outcome improves.[2]

Profiling can play a role in assessing provider performance by identifying providers who do and do not meet a certain standard of care. Utilization profiling rates for individual providers can be compared with the rate that would be expected for providers who followed an accepted practice guideline.[2]

Profiling rates may be used to make decisions about certification, credentialing, and privileging; monitoring compliance with practice guidelines and quality improvement measures; choice of physicians, hospitals, and health plans; and assessment of medical training and education.[2]

Profiling is a flexible technique for assessing provider performance. The standard of care can be based on practice guidelines (i.e., standards-based norms) or provider practice patterns (i.e., practice-based norms). Definition of acceptable performance can range from a small to a large deviation from the norm. The assessment can be focused on a single profiling rate for one condition or procedure, or it can use the results of multiple profiling rates covering a broad range of conditions or procedures. The providers being assessed may range from individual practitioner to health care organization.[2]

Profiling may make utilization review more efficient by freeing physicians from intrusive case-by-case review. Profiling can identify outliers for utilization review. Utilization profiling rates for individual physicians can be compared with rates in similar practices or with target rates based on practice guidelines. Physicians whose profiling rates differ greatly from the norm are outliers. Physician outliers can be targeted for detailed case-based review for over- or underutilization.[2]

Profiling may improve delivery of health care by the "average" physician. When a standards-based norm is available for a particular service, all profiled physicians can be notified of how their utilization profiling rates differ from the norm. Practice guidelines can be employed to encourage physicians to achieve more appropriate use of the targeted service. When standards-based norms and practice guidelines are not available, physicians in the community may review the profiling results, identify a range of appropriate utilization profiling rates, and suggest ways to achieve these rates without compromising patient outcomes.[2]

The ultimate goal of profiling is to improve health care by making medical practice more appropriate and cost-effective. To achieve this goal, profiles need to stimulate providers to review and improve their practice patterns. Profiling can reveal potential problems with the quality and the efficiency of health care delivery. Profiling can give physicians valuable information about their practice patterns and can describe how they differ from the patterns of others in terms of utilization and outcome. By exploring variation in profiling rates, physicians may learn when they are providing services that are not beneficial to patients and when they are not providing services that are. This can help physicians find ways to reduce the volume of some services without compromising the quality of patient care and to increase the volume of services (e.g., screening and preventive services) to improve patient care. Profiling can improve the efficiency and the effectiveness of utilization review by focusing on changing the behavior of the "average" physician, especially when practice guidelines and appropriate utilization and outcome rates are developed for quality assessment and quality improvement.[2]

Quality measures include both process and outcome measures. Process measures are often resource variables and may be associated with utilization profiling rates. These profiles tend to focus on compliance with standards-based norms for the care of chronic conditions, preventive services, and screening and may assess whether the recommended number of tests, procedures, or referrals occurred during a given period. For example, they may assess whether diabetic patients have a yearly glucose test and ophthalmologic visit, or whether target populations receive recommended influenza immunizations, Pap tests, and mammograms. Examples of outpatient process measures also include hospitalizations after procedures, emergency department usage, and medications prescribed. When standards-based norms have scientific justification, process measures may be considered direct measures of quality, because they reflect practice patterns shown to affect quality or quantity of life. Outcome measures are more difficult to link with specific patient-provider encounters or with a particular element of health care delivery and include variables such as mortality, morbidity, and patient functioning.[6]

Hospitals and consulting firms examine information such as final patient bills to construct profiles. One company categorizes final patient bills by diagnosis-related groups (DRGs), removes clearly unusual cases, and compares the rest with statewide or regional benchmarks based on both public and private databases. One hospital groups patients by severity of illness, categorizes resource use by diagnosis and/or physician, and compares resource utilization among hospitals. Physicians apply this resource utilization data to cut hospital costs. For example, decreased pharmacy, laboratory, and radiology charges saved an average of $2,974 on each case of gastrointestinal hemorrhage, and this program cut patient charges in general by $4.8 million in one year.[7]

Sharing Profiles with Physicians

Only recently have hospitals found it in their best interests to share such information with their physicians. This type of profiling addresses cost performance among physicians, but it does not address quality improvement issues such as compliance with practice guidelines or standards-based norms. The interests of hospitals and physicians are converging in integrated, capitated systems, because capitation means physician outliers can influence the compensation of their peers.[7]

Major changes in reimbursement systems have induced managed care organizations and hospital administrators to share physician-level information with their medical staffs. Many administrators believe information sharing is a useful tool to reduce length of stay (LOS) and ancillary resource use in order to improve financial performance under per case and per capita payment systems.[8]

Physician-level information can be shared via individual physician utilization profiles developed using patient discharge data. Development of utilization profiles requires severity adjustments, outlier removal, variance calculations, and physician scoring.[8]

One 400-bed teaching hospital reduced its LOS from 5.3 days to 4.8 days by sharing information with its medical staff, resulting in a savings of more than 7,700 patient days, or approximately 10 percent, in one year. Patients were assigned to DRGs that were categorized by severity level. Outlier cutoffs were defined, and patients with very high charges and LOS were removed. After outliers were removed, the remaining patients (inliers) were used to develop regional benchmarks for LOS and average charges within each DRG. Variances for LOS and for charges were calculated for each patient in the regional discharge data set. Variance was defined as the difference between expected and observed values based on the average for inlier patients within the region as determined by the patients' DRGs. For example, the average LOS for a low-severity, routine vaginal delivery was 1.72 for all 40,000 inlier cases in a given year. The LOS variance for a patient who stayed two days was +0.28 days (2 - 1.72). DRGs were grouped into specialty service lines to approximate the hospital's medical staff structure. For example, 40 DRGs, including vaginal deliveries and cesarean sections at all severity levels, constituted the Obstetrics Service Line. There was overlap between the orthopedic surgery and the neurosurgery departments for back surgeries; however, most DRGs fit well within service lines. Variances were calculated for each physician in the aggregate (many cases averaged together) within their service line of practice. Values were calculated per admission and per case-mix and severity-adjusted admission.[8]

Physicians were compared with other physicians in their service lines within the hospital and statewide. The individual physician was often included in multiple service lines. For example, physicians with more than 25 obstetrics cases in the year were included in the obstetrics service line; therefore, this service line included obstetricians, family practitioners, and general practitioners. Percentile rankings for resource utilization were assigned to physicians by comparing LOS and charges on a case-mix and severity-adjusted basis for physicians within their service lines across the state. A percentile ranking of 25 meant that 25 percent of physicians within that service line had lower resource utilization profiles and 75 percent had higher resource utilization profiles. The profiled physicians were benchmarked against their peers at the hospitals where they practiced, in the local competitive area, in the geographic region, and in the state.[8]

Physicians were often surprised at the variance and requested more detailed information to support their profiles. Physicians from the high end of the resource utilization scale had the strongest motivation for changing their practice patterns.[8]

Managed care organizations (MCO) are developing methods to assess the performance of their participating physicians. One MCO measured network primary care physician performance in terms of clinical results, member satisfaction, cost effectiveness, and conformance with professional/clinical standards.[9] Data on patient billing charges and hospital length of stay have been used to profile physicians and medical practices, and the profiles have been used to select or reject physicians for managed care plans and networks.[7]

Insurance claims data are often the best available source of information for MCOs to use in selecting participating physicians. Primary care physicians can be compared and selected on the basis of their resource utilization, specifically on the basis of the differences between their observed and expected use of outpatient services. Measures of resource utilization for internists included relative outpatient charges, follow-up visits, consultations, laboratory and radiology services, patient visits per year, and level of intensity of care. Using a statistical technique for risk adjustment, a prediction about the amount of resources a physician should use was developed for each measure. For example, expected laboratory use was risk-adjusted for age, gender, and case-mix; then each physician's observed use of laboratory services was compared to expected use. A pattern of care for each physician was created by comparing observed and expected resource utilization for each measure. This "profile" of differences, or pattern of variances, was used to compare physicians. Principal components analysis was used to weight the measures and to transform individual scores in the pattern of care into an overall score to permit ranking of physicians. Physicians were ranked on the basis of absolute scores obtained by summing individual scores calculated for each measure. Absolute scores indicated how far physicians differed from expectation regardless of whether the variance was positive or negative, i.e., a low revisit intensity counted against a physician in terms of variance just as much as a high revisit intensity.[9]

This study found that, while physicians differed significantly across the measures in their use of resources, adjustments made for age, gender, and case mix explained a relatively small amount of the variation in physicians' use of outpatient resources. One objection to this method of ranking was that physicians who achieved good patient outcomes with low resource use were ranked low, along with physicians who merely underutilized; thus, the method excluded some physicians who should be most sought for an MCO.[9]

The current process of credentialing physicians for managed care organizations typically verifies education, training, and work experience and then checks for the absence of negative occurrences, including malpractice claims, disciplinary actions by regulatory bodies, and loss of hospital privileges. Claims-driven "profiles" could benefit this process by adding supplementary performance-related data, such as pharmacy data, national physician claims database benchmarks, and compliance data based on the extent to which physicians' patterns of CPT-4 codes follow proprietary guidelines for appropriateness to the diagnosis.[9] "Profiles" including such information could be used as part of the initial selection process, with particular attention being paid to any resource use measures for which the physician is a significant outlier. More sophisticated "profiling" approaches can be used to evaluate the performance of physicians who are already participating in MCOs. These include comparisons of physicians' relative provision of diagnostic and preventive care, resource utilization adjusted for severity of illness and case mix, member satisfaction, and compliance with administrative rules and clinical guidelines.[9]

Resource Utilization

Competitive and financial pressures on medical practices continue to rise, and increased managed care and capitated payment systems tend to focus attention on resource allocation. Responding to market pressures, some medical practices use physician profiling as a tool to manage resource utilization (at the specialty, procedure, and diagnosis levels) within the organization and to compare physicians' practice patterns with those of their peers.[10]

In an increasingly competitive and managed care market, integration of financial, administrative, and clinical information is critical to document quality of care and lower costs through more appropriate resource utilization, more efficient use of providers, and reduction in practice variation. Resource utilization is a key determinant of health care costs. Physicians are directly or indirectly responsible for an estimated 70 percent of all health care expenditures. Medical practices need to define and to measure physician work efforts and to link these efforts with clinical practice for resource utilization management. Analysis of physician work and practice patterns involves examining the reasons for variations, such as organizational differences in systems of care, provider specialty, and patient differences. It is necessary to understand these sources of variation among physicians and practice patterns in order to compare them.[10]

There is evidence that primary care physicians use fewer resources, practice less expensive medicine, and are usually more effective than specialists in matching patients' needs and preferences with medical services. Studies have found that specialists are less accessible to patients and less oriented toward preventive medicine than to high-technology interventions. Research shows that specialists provide at least 20 percent of the primary medical care delivered in the United States, but the quality of care provided by specialists outside their specialty is declining. In addition, use of physician services differs across medical specialties and is related to patient mix. Differences in patient mix apparently explain a large part of the differences in utilization rates among organizational systems and specialty.[10]

A favorable performance assessment can be used as a marketing tool to capture managed care contracts and to negotiate advantageous reimbursement rates. Physician profiling data can also be used to contest disagreeable MCO decisions, such as erroneously branding a good physician as an outlier. Specialty medical societies have used performance assessment as a research tool to show that certain patients receive better care from a medical team directed by a specialist than from one directed by a primary care physician. Specialist societies may promote research to demonstrate that patients of specialists achieve lower morbidity and mortality, higher satisfaction and function status, and quicker return to work. The apparent result is that MCOs are increasing patient access to specialists, or what the American Medical Association (AMA) calls the "principal-care physician." National organizations are also getting involved with performance assessment and physician profiling. The National Committee for Quality Assurance (NCQA) has a Physician Organization Certification program, the Medical Group Management Association (MGMA) has a profiling system, and the AMA has the American Medical Accreditation Program (AMAP) for physician profiling. The AMA's motives in ranking physicians nationally are twofold:

■ To end the nuisance of redundant credentialing by MCOs and other organizations.

■ To take performance assessment away from MCOs and others and give it to physicians. The rationale is that, if physicians design their performance assessment system, it will be a fair evaluation that is not based solely on financial data.[4]

Most MCOs have adopted provider profiling as a means to describe provider practice patterns. In 1994, the American College of Physicians, the largest national specialty organization, issued a position paper that supported provider profiling as a valuable approach to utilization management, superior to approaches such as preauthorization of individual services.[11] Also, in 1994, an article and an editorial in the *New England Journal of Medicine* supported the concept of profiling, noting its tendency to preserve the clinical autonomy of physicians.[12] Profiling can be used to promote cost-effective care without the limitations of case-by-case preauthorization. True clinical profiling, using episode of care methodology and practice benchmarks, can supply providers with data to review and alter practice patterns.[11]

Profiling has been defined as a description of disease-specific practice patterns and comparison of these patterns to an appropriate peer group in order to establish practice benchmarks. There is evidence that a few "best practice" and many cost-effective strategies for health care can be identified for specific diseases and that there is substantial practice variation among providers around these strategies that are not explained by demographics or patient characteristics.[11]

Another approach to profiling involves analysis of episodes of care, or clinical "units" created from claims or encounter data, especially for acute and subacute care. The beginning and the ending of the episode are identified, and related diagnoses are linked in Episode Treatment Groups (ETGs) analogous to hospital-based DRGs. ETGs consist of primary diagnoses involving similar clinical management and incorporate care at any site. If both cost and clinical issues are being considered, episodes are compared instead of analyzing care over a time interval. Comparison of episodes allows differentiation of patients who may have only one episode in an interval from patients with multiple episodes. ETGs can also be used to evaluate case mix. Unlike resource-derived systems and regression-based methods that link unrelated diagnoses based largely on resource use, a clinically based system involving ETGs can be used to adjust for case mix within a specific clinical area (e.g., renal disease) or a specific specialty (e.g., urology).[11]

The Evolution of Profiling

Increasingly, physicians in the United States are practicing in groups, and most, if not all, group practices are involved in managed care. Large, multispecialty physician group practices can use physician profiling to monitor and improve quality and efficiency. Groups can measure physician performance by examining ratios of medical inputs to patient population outputs.[1]

Physician profiling focuses on patterns of care rather than on individual occurrences of care and generally uses large, computerized databases. Profiles are usually expressed as a ratio of inputs and outputs and vary in their complexity. The ratios measure utilization or outcome aggregated over time for a specific population of patients under the care of a provider or group of providers. A simple profile may express the number of claims for a specific procedure that a physician submits per year (a measure of input) across all of that physician's patients (a measure of output). A more complex profile may express the number of specific diagnostic tests performed as indicated by practice guidelines for patients with a certain condition.[1]

Originally, profiling was simple and focused at the hospital, acute care episode level and was extended to outpatient care as hospital utilization decreased. This initial profiling involved analyzing patterns of care by counting the numbers and intensity of services rendered in aggregate terms. Current profiling includes more of the patient's complete medical condition. Profiles often go beyond tallying the resources used at a given time (an inpatient admission or an outpatient visit) to overall resource utilization precipitated by the patient's contact with the health care delivery system.[1]

Profiles may link resource utilization to specific conditions that are relevant to a particular patient population. Inpatient measures may include length of stay, number of procedures, and resource use (e.g., laboratory tests). Outpatient measures may include number of patients seen per period, number of procedures performed, and resource use. Profiles may include patient satisfaction surveys and quality of care as measured by adherence to practice guidelines. The use of patient outcome measures for profiling is limited by the rare occurrence of seriously bad outcomes, incomplete understanding of risk factors, patient preferences, multiple causes for functional impairment, and long periods until poor outcomes appear.[1]

Typically, the goals of physician profiling are to lower the cost of patient care and/or to improve the quality of patient care. Group medical practices can use profiling to achieve these goals by:

- Sharing profiles with individual physicians to foster behavioral change.

- Linking profiles to physician compensation as a financial incentive.

- Using profile statistics in contract negotiations with payers.

- Distinguishing between individual and systemic factors in utilization review.

- Monitoring the quality of patient care for capitated plans.[1]

Insurers and managed care organizations typically use claims data to identify physicians who consistently use more resources than their peers. Providers with expensive practice patterns are penalized financially or dropped from the provider network. Managed care organizations may reward efficient providers whose patterns fall within established norms by selecting them for preferred provider networks or bypassing the requirement for detailed case-by-case review. In 1992, 45.5 percent of physicians were subject to clinical or economic profiling, yet less than half of them received feedback regularly.[1]

As well-trained scientists, physicians can understand the value of information and can respond to valid and useful data about their practice patterns. Group practices can use consensus to develop and implement profiles based on group norms and guidelines in order to track trends and make systemic changes in a timely fashion. Profiling can give a group practice a competitive advantage by providing timely information to aid in strategic planning for practice management, including diagnostic testing, vendor use, and clinic administration.[1]

A basic level of resource utilization profiling would report a ratio, such as average cost per hip replacement for orthopedic surgeons, and identify those who lie outside the norm. The next level of profiling may determine that this variance is due to the hospital's inefficient purchasing policy regarding prostheses and lead to a change in hospital policy to allow for competitive bidding for high-cost medical equipment. Ultimately, profiling information on appropriateness of surgery, use of ancillaries, and patient outcomes (postoperative morbidity and recovery, functional status, satisfaction, and quality of life) can influence physicians' behavior.[1]

Reducing practice variation can save time and increase patient throughput in an emergency department. Health care providers who are at financial risk for the cost of care need a method to monitor and manage that risk. Emergency physicians used practice profiling with practice guidelines to reduce the annualized cost of 30,000 emergency department visits at one hospital by $31.32 per patient visit, or $939,600.[13]

Physician profiling may be used to align the demand for, and supply of, primary care physician time. Physician profiling can be adapted to manage primary care panels systems in MCOs and can be applied to: allocating primary care physician staff to clinics, determining which panels to open and which to close to new enrollment, and estimating how to compensate primary care physicians.[14]

Patients, physicians, and payers can benefit from efficient use of resources and from strategies to improve the alignment of demand for primary care physician time with supply of primary care physician time in MCOs. Patient access problems can lead to enrollee dissatisfaction and turnover in MCO enrollment. Physician dissatisfaction with case-mix adjustment for panel populations and their compensation can lead to physician staff turnover. Efficient use of resources can help MCOs maintain a competitive advantage in the marketplace.[14]

Case mix information has been used to generate measures of panel case complexity and physician practice style (numbers of progress visits and specialist referrals) for primary care and for specialist care. A profiling ratio called "practice style factor" (PSF) is the ratio of observed visits accrued to a panel and the expected visits estimated for the panel population adjusted for case complexity. Practice style is used to suggest how primary care physicians manage demand for primary care time on their panels. An MCO may interpret the ratio of observed to estimated primary care visits as the extent to which a primary care physician has managed a panel population regarding visits and referrals to specialists. An MCO may apply this physician profiling method to the design and management of primary care panels. The goal is to support resource allocation strategies: allocation of primary care physician time, determination of which panels to open or close to new enrollment, and adjustment of physician compensation to pay for varying workloads.[14]

There is evidence of variations in cost and utilization across communities, and patient populations differ in their clinical characteristics. Physician profiles use statistical techniques known as risk adjustment to account for relevant patient characteristics before making inferences about the effectiveness of care.[15]

Medicare

Primary care practices in three states representing different regions of the country were profiled using claims data from the Health Care Financing

Administration's (HCFA) National Claims History File (NCHF) from 1990 to 1991 for Medicare beneficiaries. As expected, practice profiles showed that practices with sicker patients were found to be more expensive than practices with healthier patients and that older patients consume more financial resources than younger patients. Significant variation in use and cost exists among different primary care practice types. Internal medicine and group practices were associated with higher per patient resource use. Differences in provider efficiency and sicker patients may explain this finding. Smaller practices were associated with higher rates of service use and cost. Large practices were associated with less use of hospital services. Small practices were associated with higher ambulatory service use. These results suggest that patients managed by smaller practices may require more intensive treatment, but there was little evidence that smaller practices were seeing sicker patients. The study results could not explain why smaller practices were more resource intensive than large practices. Patient case-mix characteristics were an important component of profiling Medicare primary care practices. Health service use and cost increased with patient age. Age and gender, however, were not associated with laboratory use, and gender had less effect on ambulatory visits than it did on use of hospital services. Males received more medical care than females; perhaps males delayed going to physicians until their medical problems became significant.[16]

This study offered several health policy implications. Health care organizations seeking to enter the Medicare managed care market can construct office-based practice profiles for fee-for-service Medicare beneficiaries. Health care organizations can profile their panels of practices serving Medicare contracts to monitor utilization and cost differences. Profiling primary care practices acting as gatekeepers can provide vital information for managed care organizations entering the Medicare market, especially if they intend to rely on some fee-for-service transactions for enrollees to opt out of an existing network of providers. The legislation requiring Medicare managed care organizations to provide transaction-level claims data or some equivalent (e.g., episode-of-care data) to HCFA makes such comprehensive practice profiles possible.[16]

This study demonstrates the creation of practice profiles of office-based providers serving fee-for-service Medicare beneficiaries. It illustrates the use of fee-for-service claims to examine systematic differences in health care utilization and cost. Profiling all implicit gatekeepers for several hundred thousand Medicare beneficiaries in Alabama, Iowa, and Maryland showed significant differences in health care resource use by specialty, practice size, and group practice configuration. In this study, family practitioners used fewer resources than internists and multispecialty group practices, and larger practices were less costly than smaller practices, after controlling for practice case mix and metropolitan location.[16]

Physician profiles can provide managed care organizations with information to improve the efficiency and quality of health care delivered. Practice profiles created from public use data sources can provide valuable strategic information to health care organizations and policy makers as the Medicare managed care market develops.[16]

References

1. Tompkins, C., and others. "Physician Profiling in Group Practices." *Journal of Ambulatory Care Management* 19(4):28-39, Oct. 1996.

2. Lasker, R., and others. "Realizing the Potential of Practice Pattern Profiling." *Inquiry* 29(3):287-97, Fall 1992.

3. Ruffin, M. "Physician Profiling: Trends and Implications." *Physician Executive* 21(11):34-7, Nov. 1995.

4. Pretzer, M. "Physician Profiling Can Work in Your Favor." *Medical Economics* 74(12): 51-2,55,58, June 9, 1997.

5. Lauve, R. "Rationale for Physician Profiling Explained." *Physician's Management* 37(1):29-31, Jan. 1, 1997.

6. McNeil, B., and others. "Current Issues in Profiling Quality of Care." *Inquiry* 29(3):298-307, Fall 1992.

7. Montague, J. "Profiling in Practice." *Hospitals & Health Networks* 68(2):50-1, Jan. 20, 1994.

8. Bennett, G., and others. "Case Study in Physician Profiling." *Managed Care Quarterly* 2(4):60-70, Autumn 1994.

9. Nathanson, P., and others. "Using Claims Data to Select Primary Care Physicians for a Managed Care Network." *Managed Care Quarterly* 2(4):50-9, Autumn 1994.

10. Newman, C., and others. "Physician Profiling: Applications for the Robert Wood Johnson Profiling Project Database." *Journal of Ambulatory Care Management* 19(4):49-57, Oct. 1996.

11. Miller, L. "Provider Profiling: Advancing to Episodes of Care." *Physician Executive* 21(10):40-1, Oct. 1995.

12. Welch, G., and others. "Physician Profiling: An Analysis of Inpatient Practice Patterns in Florida and Oregon." *New England Journal of Medicine* 330(9):607-12, March 3, 1994.

13. Ahwah, I., and Karpiel, M. "Using Profiling for Cost and Quality Management in the Emergency Department." *Healthcare Financial Management* 51(7):48,50-3, July 1997.

14. Roblin, D. "Applications of Physician Profiling in the Management of Primary Care Panels." *Journal of Ambulatory Care Management* 19(2):59-74, April 1996.

15. Chang, W., and McCracken, S. "Applying Case Mix Adjustment in Profiling Primary Care Physician Performance." *Journal of Health Care Finance* 22(4):1-9, Summer 1996.

16. Parente, S., and others. "Profiling Resource Use by Primary-Care Practices: Managed Medicare Implications." *Health Care Financing Review* 17(4):23-42, Summer 1996.

Marilyn Szymialis Radke, MD, MPH, MA, FACPM, CPE, FACPE, was Medical Officer, Drug Enforcement Administration, Arlington, Virginia, when this chapter was written. She is now a clinical fellow in occupational and environmental medicine at Johns Hopkins University School of Medicine, Baltimore, Maryland.

SECTION II

Issues and Concerns in Physician Profiling

CHAPTER 3

Elements of a Physician Profile
by Jonathan Bogen, MSPH, MBA, CHE

*T*he purpose of this chapter is to familiarize the reader with key elements of a profile, sources of variation, and profiling techniques and formats. The importance of case-mix measurement will be discussed and various methods will be examined. Finally, an overview of basic medical statistics is presented and related to methods used for provider profiles.

Overview

The general purpose of provider profiling is to evaluate variation in practice patterns and to provide feedback to providers. Physician profiles report simple process quality measures, utilization rates of tests and referrals, and patient-associated charges. Profiles should not be based on a black-box approach. They should be open to inspection as to the methodology used and the rationale for acceptable variation.

Some form of risk adjustment is always necessary in provider profiles. Traditional actuarial models use demographic factors (e.g., age, sex, and town of residence) in health insurance underwriting. Risk adjustment makes sure that providers who treat high-risk patients are not penalized.

Physician profiles should be grounded in proper statistical and clinical methodology. The information displayed should be clear and should allow for timely follow-up. Most profiles should allow roll-ups into larger major categories for comparison and drill down into smaller and smaller subcategories for further analysis. Generally, profiles are developed from administrative data (e.g., claims, encounter data, hospital information system, etc.). The advantage of profiling administrative data is low cost, because the data are already collected for billing purposes. However, the data are not clinically rich and may not always be an accurate representation of the clinical condition of the patient. Important methodological issues in profiling are the accuracy of the administrative data or other data sources, edits to the data set, and sampling error.

Edits

In collecting data for physician profiles, one must first develop a set of edits to account for missing data, outliers, or mis-coded data. Outliers are data values beyond the normal range of values and may represent data errors or unusual values. Nevertheless, one must decide to leave outliers in or out. For instance, length of stay outliers can be the result of invalid admission or discharge dates, early discharge (i.e., discharged before midnight), or special circumstances in which the patient cannot be discharged. Edits can be based on outlier values far outside the normal range of values or validity edits (e.g., mismatched diagnoses based on age or sex). The decision to remove outliers may be based on a combination of statistical, clinical, and health policy considerations. Because utilization data tend not to be normally distributed, the statistically inclined opt for a lognormal transformation to trim outliers, while others use a combination of standard deviation or percentiles. All statistical software routinely produces descriptive statistics used to identify outliers and to develop trim points (see sample data output in table 1, below).[1] The standard deviation and the variance tell us about the variability or spread of sample data from the mean. Skewness and kurtosis tell us about the distribution of the data according to a normal or "bell shaped" curve.

TABLE 1. SAMPLE OUTPUT FOR A PATIENT LENGTH OF STAY IN A REHABILITATION HOSPITAL[1]

Number of Cases	Min. Value	Max. Value	Mean (ALOS)	Standard Deviation	Variance	Skewness	Kurtosis
2,087	3.00	264.00	23.58	18.63	347.04	3.45	26.11
Note	*All values, except for cases, are in days.*						

Validity edits can be quite extensive, and a number of software products have been developed to compare data elements of a UB-92 or HCFA-1500 claim for validity. For example, how does one handle maternity claims where mother and infant have the same claim record? A more difficult process is handling inaccurate diagnostic or procedure coding, which is critical to determining case mix and reimbursement. In this case, it is wise to take a systematic sample of administrative data and compare the coded data to the medical charts for accuracy. Conducting coding audits of sampled data records can serve to validate unusual practice patterns. Published studies have generally reported a wide variation in diagnostic coding accuracy. Under capitated reimbursement, many usual data elements may be entirely missing or incomplete. Therefore, one needs to develop procedures to deal with the issue of missing data, such as which records to trim from the profile. Under capitation, the only data source for profiling may be the medical chart or encounter data.

Sampling Error

Because of cost or resource issues, it may be necessary to collect sample data for provider profiles. Generally, the statistical population is preferred, but sampling is acceptable when performed correctly. One must guard against Type I and Type II error when sampling data. Type I error (α) is declaring a real difference exists between two rates when the difference is in fact zero. A Type II error (() consists of not finding a difference that actually exists between two rates. Type II error can be controlled by specifying the Power of the test $(1-\beta)$.[2] Most statistical software will calculate sample sizes based on specifying a combination of (and power $(1-\beta)$; alternatively, sample size tables or power curve diagrams could be used.

Elements of a Profile

The data elements of physician profiles differ, depending on the purpose and the setting-e.g., if the purpose is to track practice pattern variation, identify cost outliers, or identify physicians for withholds or bonuses. For providers that have risk or capitated arrangements, the profile might be weighted more to financial or utilization measures and used by the payer to determine bonus points or incentives for providers based on utilization targets. For credentialing within a hospital, quality of care measures might be more applicable, or a utilization review department will naturally be interested in utilization profiles.

Generally, physician profiles fall into four categories:

■ Utilization and cost data.

■ Quality of care indicators.

■ Access.

■ Patient satisfaction.

Utilization and cost data are the most commonly generated physician profiles, although more primary care physicians are receiving HEDIS profiles of their quality of care. Everyone in medicine since the advent of managed care is now familiar with the PMPM (per member per month) initialism. For practice management, providers and payers need to know how much is being spent for each member for each month. Because the medical loss ratio (i.e., how much is actually spent on providing patient care services) and the requirement for medical claims reserves (due to IBNR) need to be budgeted, actual PMPM versus expected PMPM is generally useful. (IBNR, or "incurred but not reported," refers to any outstanding medical claims that have not been billed or fully adjudicated by the insurer.) Higher than expected PMPM indicates that volume, cost, or intensity of services is increased. Another area of concern is prescription drug charges, so profiles tracking associated pharmacy costs by physician may be useful, especially where a formulary is used.

Members versus Patients

The goal in medicine today is no longer to simply treat disease but to improve the health status of the community. Tracking members as opposed to patients is an important conceptual change. Under managed care, primary care physicians (PCP) are expected to ensure that members are provided appropriate medical care in the right setting at the right time. Member level data are possible because patients are assigned to particular provider panels and members' utilization is apportioned to particular providers. Because, in fee-for-service medicine, patients may be under the care of multiple providers without the guidance of a PCP, only patient-level tracking is practical. For specialists, profiles track patient-level data only. Generally, membership is reported on a member-month basis. To compute member months, one multiplies the number of patient/members by the number of months they have been patients. Even under fee-for-service arrangements, patients can be tracked as members with assigned start and end dates in the practice management or hospital billing system. In the absence of start and end dates, an estimate of member months can be used.

Rates versus Ratios

Profile data can be reported as frequencies (e.g., number of ECGs by provider), percentages (e.g., percent of patients extremely satisfied with care), or averages (ALOS, or average length of stay). To be able to compare providers and monitor variation, rates and ratios are necessary. PMPM is an example of a common rate. Rates are reported to control (i.e., standardize) for the size of the membership. One would not compare payments to providers without accounting for the number of members assigned to each provider.

For the average physician or health care manager, these types of profiles are difficult to interpret in terms of assessing provider performance. Most useful to the provider or the manager is information on whether the provider is better or worse than some accepted benchmark. Therefore, provider profiles should use ratios or statistical tests for significance to compare the indicator being profiled to the expected value. The expected rates can be based on a set standard or on a comparison against the case-mix adjusted rate. Most often, comparison of actual rates to expected rates is given by a ratio (observed value/expected value), which is analogous to relative risk (RR). The odds ratio or risk ratio are sometimes computed as well. For example, a ratio of 1.25 of observed to expected value implies that the provider is 25 percent better than expected and a ratio of .75 implies that the provider is 25 percent worse than expected. The ratio should be employed only with sufficient sample size (i.e., at least 25 cases) and confidence limits around the ratio or whether the difference is statistically significant should always be indicated. Fewer cases result in wider confidence limits, and a large number of cases shortens the confidence limits, resulting in greater precision (i.e., the ability to determine that a statistical difference exists in the rates).[3] Sample profile measures and indicators are shown in table 2, page 42-43.

Reasons for Variation in Physician Profiles

Utilization rates are influenced by a number of factors, including volume, case mix, health status, costs and intensity of services, and size of membership. Physicians treating more high-cost cases or a large number of members with chronic symptoms will naturally have higher costs and utilization associated with those patients. When reviewing profiles, one should ask the following questions:

■ What time period was profiled.

■ If a sample of records was profiled, how was the sample chosen and what size sample was used.

■ What case-mix method was used for risk adjustment.

Risk Adjustment

Generally, in the use of physician practice profiles, one hopes to develop measures that are both clinically and statistically valid. As we already discussed, some case-mix or severity adjustment is necessary if useful comparisons are to be made.

Risk adjustment is a technique generally used in standardizing utilization rates, morbidity, and mortality rates based on patient case mix. Case mix can be defined in a number of ways, including demographic factors (e.g., age, sex, residence), diagnoses (type and range of diagnoses and procedure codes), and severity of illness (health status and comorbidities). For example, mortality rates at tertiary care hospitals would not be compared with mortality rates at community hospitals without some form of risk adjustment. In fact, public release by HCFA of hospital mortality rates for Medicare patients was shelved after it received extensive criticism for the method of risk adjustment used. A typical risk-adjustment model might include various risk factors, such as diagnosis, age,

TABLE 2. SAMPLE PROFILE MEASURES AND INDICATORS

Measure	Units of Measure	How Computed
I. UTILIZATION		
Admission Rate	Admits	(Total admissions/MM) x 12 x 1000
Days rate	Days	(Total hospital days/MM) x 12 x 1000
Average length of stay.	Average in days	Total hospital days/Number of admissions
Outpatient visit rate.	Proportional rate	(Total encounters/MM) x 12 x 1000
C-section rate.	Percentage	(Total C-section/deliveries) x 100%
Surgical case rate	Proportional rate	(Total surgical cases/MM) x 12 x 1000
Readmission rate within 90 days.	Proportional rate	(Total readmissions/all admits) x 1000
Lab test rate	Proportional rate	(Total labs/MM) x 12 x 1000
Radiology rate	Proportional rate	(Total radiographs/MM) x 12 x 1000
Number of outpatient services per visit.	Proportional rate	(Total outpatient ancillaries/MM) x 12 x 1000
Specialist referral rate	Proportional rate	(Total specialty visits/members) x 12 x 1000
Payment rate (PMPM)	Total dollars paid	(Total reimbursements /MM) x 12 x 1000
Average payments/encounter.	Average dollars	Total reimbursements/total encounters
Cost per member per month (PMPM).	Average dollars	(Total payments/MM) x 12 x 1000
Prescription cost (PMPM)	Average dollars	Total prescription payments/MM
Non-formulary use	Percentage	(Total prescriptions off formulary/all prescriptions) x 100%
II. QUALITY		
Diabetic eye exam rate	Proportional Screening rate	Number of patients with retinal eye exams/number of diabetic patients
Mammography screening rate	Proportional Screening rate	Number of females with mammograms/PAR
Pap smear rate	Proportional Screening rate	Number of females with Pap tests/PAR
Complication rate/100.	Percent	Number of surgical patients with complications/surgical patients x 100%
Return to OR	Percent	(Number of surgical patients with unscheduled OR procedures/surgical patients) x 100%
Functional health status	Average	Health status average score
Mortality rate	Rate	(Number of patients who died/all patients) x 1000

TABLE 2. SAMPLE PROFILE MEASURES AND INDICATORS (CONT'D)

Measure	Units of Measure	How Computed
III. ACCESS/AVAILABILITY		
Waiting time for new appointment.	Average	Total wait times/number of new appointments
Patient turnover/100.	Percent	Number of disenrolled patients/all patients in two-year time period
Out of plan referrals/1000.	Proportional rate	(Number of out-of-plan referrals/MM) x 12 x 1000
Emergency department (ED) encounters /1000.	Proportional rate	(Number of ED encounters/MM) x 12 1000
IV. SATISFACTION		
Dissatisfied Percentage	Percent	(Number of patient dissatisfied/all patient) x 100%

Notes:

1. Member months (MM): sum of months for each enrollee tabulated each quarter or per annual period.

2. Annual rates involving MM are multiplied by 12 (months) and 1000 to express in MM. Note, for rates involving MM on a quarterly or biannual period, multiply by a factor of 3 or 6 (months), respectively

3. Days of Care Rate =Discharge Rate x ALOS

4. Proportional rates are expressed in a per 1000 rate or a per 100 rate in order to express the result of the division as an integer. Note, a per 100 rate is equal to a percentage.

5. PAR: Population-at-risk. For mammography or PAP test, it varies according to specific age guidelines for women.

6. Encounters may be based on multiple visits if billed together.

7. Generally insurance actual payments are used instead of dollar charges for PMPM unless otherwise noted. Payments do not factor in discounts, copayments, and other deductibles in comparing PMPM or other payment based rate.

gender, and presence of chronic disease conditions. Choosing the method of risk adjustment is an important decision that might ultimately be based on a number of factors, including data quality. The ultimate goal is to account for variability in outcomes based on patient factors not under the direct control of the physician. Once patient factors are accounted for, the data can be used to assess the effects of provider practice patterns, chance, and other unexplained factors on performance measures.

Some risk-adjustment methods use clinical data that must be specifically coded or abstracted from medical records. Other risk-adjustment methods use administrative data or claims-based information. No risk-adjustment model should be used without proper testing to determine its validity and reliability. Validity corresponds to the clinical plausibility of the model and to its success in grouping clinically similar cases. Reliability is based on the statistical ability of the model to obtain similar results with repeated sampling.

Risk-adjustment methods are also employed in actuarial or reimbursement models to predict utilization and cost of health resources. While traditional health insurance underwriting includes age, sex, and residence, prospective reimbursement requires risk-adjustment factors such as diagnosis, presence of chronic conditions, and health status. Risk adjustment is important to PCPs who practice under managed care because capitation rates depend on their case mix.

Inpatient Case Mix Measures

Diagnosis-related groups (DRGs) are probably the most universally used measure of case mix. Medicare has come up with 490 distinct DRGs, and the AP-DRGs (all-payer diagnosis-related groups) include additional DRGs for pediatric and HIV-related illness. Research on case mix, which was originally designed for the development of prospective reimbursement systems, has been largely funded by the HCFA but has been adopted by private payers.

Many methods of determining case mix have been criticized for failing to measure severity of illness. For example, patients in DRG 88 (chronic obstructive pulmonary disease) may differ in health status and functional ability. Ideally, a measure of comorbidity, functional status, or disability should be included in the case-mix assessment. Various measures of severity of illness have been developed: APR-DRGs (All Patient Refined Diagnosis-Related Groups), disease staging methods (where patients are scored from 1 to 5, depending on their stage of illness), patient management categories (PMCs), MedisGroups, and acute physiology and chronic health evaluations (APACHEs). The first three-APR-DRGs, disease staging methods, and PMCs-use administrative data. The latter two require clinical data from medical chart review. According to a recent report, severity-of-illness measures produced different results, depending on the diagnostic group. This led the author of the study to conclude that "severity-adjusted mortality rates alone are unlikely to isolate quality differences across hospitals."[4]

Episode-Level Case-Mix Measures

A number of case-mix measurement systems combine ambulatory and inpatient visits into clinically related encounters. For instance, ambulatory care groups (ACGs) developed at John Hopkins University utilize up to 52 ACGs for risk adjustment. Similar visits are grouped into episodes of care, which means, for example, that a diabetic patient's inpatient and outpatient visits would all be considered part of one ACG. Thirty-four ADGs (Ambulatory Diagnostic Groups) are the building blocks of 52 ACGs. Some payers use ACGs to profile utilization rates and charges. In a study of capitation models that had been designed to predict health care resource utilization of health maintenance organization (HMO) members ages 18 to 64, models that used self-reported health status plus diagnosis were better at predicting future resource utilization than were models based only on demographic factors.[5] For primary care providers who treat many chronic disease patients, diagnostic risk-adjustment models are important in terms of case management. DCGs (Diagnostic Cost Groups) are another severity-of-illness method used to adjust patient data into clinically and statistically valid case mix groupings. The DCG model predicts medical costs by identifying a patient's costliest diagnosis.[6] Medicare has indicated its intention of utilizing PIP-DCGs (Principal Inpatient Procedure-Diagnostic Cost Groups) for setting PSO and Medicare HMO rates under the Medicare + Choice Program. Another episode-level case-mix method, Episode Treatment Groups (ETGs), combines ambulatory and inpatient claims into 558 treatment episodes. Generally, most episode grouper systems utilize a fixed period to create episodes; ETGs vary by episode.

The Society of Actuaries' Health Risk Adjustment Study assessed the various risk-adjustment methods for both predicting future health utilization and explaining past or historical utilization.[7] The validity and reliability of risk-adjustment models are determined primarily in two ways-reduction in variability and predictive power. For predicting medical expenses for a group of patients, age/sex alone was almost as good a predictor as the other three case-mix models (i.e., low predictive error). Risk adjustment that uses diagnostic information on medical claims to adjust payments generally appears to provide the best ability to predict future patient costs. Without a reliable risk-adjustment model, it is likely that capitation rates will either over- or under-pay physicians.

Types of Provider Profiles
Statistical Process Measures

The total quality management (TQM) movement adapted from industrial quality control methods has been embraced by the health care industry. The underpinning of TQM or CQI (continuous quality improvement) is statistical process control, which is a set of statistical techniques used to measure processes that are in or out of control. Pioneers in the application of TQM methods included Walter Shewhart, W.E. Deming, J.M. Juran, Philip Crosby, and others. The most common control charts used to determine whether a process is in control are P-charts, X-Bar charts, or R-charts. (For an excellent primer on the use of control charts in health care improvement, see Berwick *et al.*[8]) The P-chart is used for measures, such as mortality, infection rates, complications, etc., that can be described using a normal probability distribution X-Bar charts are generally used for ordinal data, such as length of stay, number of tests, waiting time, etc. A sample X-Bar chart for average length of stay at a rehabilitation hospital is shown in the figure below, with months represented on the X-axis and the ALOS in days on the Y-axis. The upper control limit (UCL) and lower control limit (LCL) are shown as well. The chart actually indicated a data problem with capturing patient days, rather than a steady increase in ALOS over the course of the year. A "special cause" variation is noted in January and February because of an error by a billing clerk.

X-BAR CHART FOR AVERAGE LENGTH OF STAY BY MONTH
X-BAR Chart for ALOS by Month

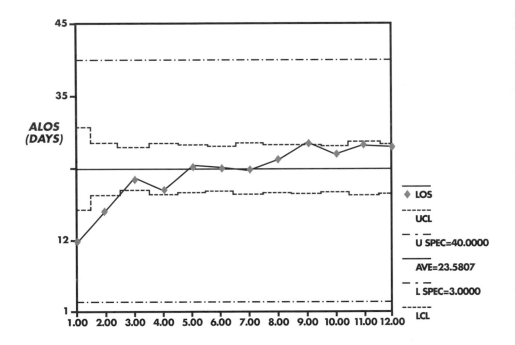

Benchmarking
Along with TQM, benchmarking is increasingly being used in health care to foster performance improvement. Benchmarking consists of deciding what constitutes best practice and comparing one's rate to that standard. For example, an institution might want to reduce the incidence of non-emergency cases treated in the emergency department. It might compare its rate to that of a similar facility or set a standard based on reducing the proportion of non-emergency or urgent diagnoses treated in the emergency department.

Most commercial profiling tools provide benchmarks. Benchmark data are available from public and private specialty societies, NCQA (Quality Compass), and federal agencies (USPHS, AHCPR, HCFA).

Health Employer Data and Information Set (HEDIS)

Managed care organizations (MCOs) are at the forefront of a relatively new trend, using provider report cards to profile providers and to ensure compliance with various standards and guidelines. To receive NCQA accreditation, an MCO must have data systems that can capture Health Employer Data and Information Set (HEDIS) data. HEDIS is one of many attempts to standardize the measurement of quality of care by MCOs. HEDIS was developed as a set of performance measures to compare managed care health plans. Originally, HEDIS included only process measures of performance, but the latest version, HEDIS 3.0, also incorporates some outcome measures.

Large health insurance (employer) purchasing coalitions are using HEDIS measures to compare the performance of health plans. NCQA's Quality Compass is a national database of comparative information that can be used to evaluate the quality of managed care plans. However, consumers have indicated that the measures are not useful to them in differentiating among health plans. In general, consumers seem to prefer measures of satisfaction.

Health plans that fall below desired rates are expected to profile their PCPs intensively to increase performance rates. Physicians can be profiled by their group practices, by the hospitals with which they are affiliated, or individually using screening or best practice rates as benchmarks. Because patients must choose a PCP when initially enrolled in an MCO, it is possible to compute the number of patients per physician panel that meet the HEDIS criteria (e.g., population-at-risk and number of patients meeting the guidelines).

A large MCO with approximately 262,000 contracted physicians has begun to send its physicians reports of their performance on six HEDIS-like clinical measures.[9] For example, how many patients received beta blockers after acute myocardial infarction? How many patients with diabetes received glycated hemoglobin tests? Most health plans do not routinely use these measures for profiling providers because the sample size of provider panels is too small for statistically valid comparisons. Nevertheless, in some hospital-based group practices, the patient panel may be large enough to profile HEDIS rates by medical group hospital affiliation.

The proponents of HEDIS and similar report cards see them as a means to further population-based medicine. However, there are problems with these report cards. For example, how do you define accountability at the provider level, especially when a provider with multiple insurer contracts is being profiled on a selected sample basis (i.e., not population based)? In addition, for individual providers to undertake measurement studies, a stable patient panel for at least two years is mandatory.

How Are HEDIS Rates Computed?

In profiling a population of MCO members, the underlying population-at-risk (PAR) needs to be determined. From an epidemiological perspective, PAR varies by disease. For example, to study prenatal care, the population-at-risk is women of childbearing years. In computing the HEDIS rate, the denominator represents a systematic sample of the plan's PAR; the numerator represents the number of patients in this group who have received the health care service (see example below).

Sample Indicator: Mammography Screening Rate for Non-Medicare Members.[10] This is the percentage of women ages 52 to 64 who had mammograms in the previous two years.

Numerator. This is the number of women in the denominator who had a mammogram in the two-year period.

Denominator. This is the number of women ages 52 to 64 inclusive who were continuously enrolled during the two-year period. (Note: Continuous enrollment means that the women belonged to the same MCO for the entire two-year period, with no more than a 60-day break in membership. Also, the patients must have remained with the same physician group for the entire period. If patients did not stay with the same group during this period, an estimate of member months may be permitted. Continuous enrollment is used to compensate for turnover when members switch health plans.)

Data Source. The data source for the numerator should include audited evidence that the patient had a mammogram during the two-year period, e.g., a paid claim for a mammogram or the number of female patients or a clinical note for a mammogram. If a claim is not found, a medical chart review is required.

Public Provider Profiles

Various public efforts are under way to produce report cards that evaluate the performance of providers (i.e., hospitals or physicians). Notable efforts include the public release by New York and Pennsylvania of mortality data for coronary artery bypass grafting (CABG). New York and Pennsylvania were actually mandated by their state legislatures to release these data. Pennsylvania used MedisGroups for risk adjustment; New York used its own diagnosis-related model. The Pennsylvania effort has been criticized, because the annual volume of CABG surgeries performed in the state may be too small for meaningful comparisons among physicians.

Cleveland's Health Quality Choice Coalition publishes comparisons of Cleveland's hospitals every six months.[11] The comparisons utilize severity and case-mix adjustment, so that comparative reports describe a hospital's performance above or below predicted levels. Employers reported that they wanted price information as well as key outcomes on hospitals. Employers were interested in the functional status of patients after surgery. For example, what is the health status of diabetics? How many emergency department visits and costs were incurred for this disease population? Other quality indicators include patient satisfaction, in-hospital mortality, and hospital-acquired complications. Consumers wanted information on physician and hospital performance.

Conclusion

The Pennsylvania Corporate Hospital Rating Project found that the strongest demand from corporate benefit managers was for profiles to rate individual physicians or physician groups.[12] From a provider perspective, it will be increasingly important to develop practice profiles that both ensure and improve quality of care. As we have seen, provider profiling has traditionally focused only at the hospital or health plan level. However, there is increasing desire on the part of insurers and employers alike to obtain useful report cards on physicians. Because physician profiles are difficult for the average consumer to interpret, consumers are more interested in obtaining patient satisfaction information on physicians. Patient satisfaction information is rarely collected by physicians or medical groups, although various innovative surveys have been attempted.

Because provider report cards and capitation are not likely to disappear anytime soon, PCPs will need to develop internal reporting systems to report HEDIS-type data and to monitor utilization. HEDIS measures are publicly available, and medical groups can use them in benchmarking. Prior utilization has a relatively high predictive power, but validity and reliability depend on the accuracy of the coded diagnostic information. With the increasing emphasis on capitation, the burden will be on the PCP to report these data, because important data will be absent in the professional claim. Some practice management systems already have this capability. However, the development of better systems to capture patient enrollment data and merge them with clinical data will help immensely in streamlining a process that should ultimately become routine.

References

1. SPSS for Windows, Release 7.0, Standard Version, SPSS, Inc., Chicago, Ill., 1989-1995.

2. Fleiss, J. *Statistical Methods for Rates and Proportions*, Second Edition. New York, N.Y.: John Wiley & Sons,1981.

3. Norusis, M. *The SPSS Guide to Data Analysis*. Chicago, Ill.: SPSS, Inc., 1986.

4. Iezzoni, L. "The Risks of Risk Adjustment." *JAMA* 278(19):1600-7, Nov. 19, 1997.

5. Fowles, J., and others. "Taking Health Status into Account When Setting Capitation Rates." *JAMA* 276(16):1316-1321, Oct. 23-30, 1996.

6. Ellis, R., and others. "Diagnosis-Based Risk Adjustment for Medicare Capitation Payments." *Health Care Financing Review* 17(3):101-28, Spring 1996.

7. Dunn, D., and others. *A Comparative Analysis of Methods of Health Risk Assessment*, M-HB96-1. Schaumburg, Ill.: Society of Actuaries, Oct. 1996.

8. Berwick, D., and others. *Curing Health Care—New Strategies for Quality Improvement*. San Francsico, Calif.: Jossey-Bass, 1990.

9. "One-Page Profile Shows Physicians How Practice Patterns Stack Up Against Standards." *Data Strategies and Benchmarks*. 2(1):13-5, Jan. 1998.

10. NCQA HEDIS Version 3.0/1998, Addendum. Washington, DC: National Committee for Quality Assurance, 1998.

11. Harper, D. "The Cleveland Project: Reporting on Quality." *Healthcare Executive* 13(3):68-9, May/June 1998.

12. Pauly, M., and others. "Measuring Hospital Outcomes from a Buyer's Perspective." *American Journal of Medical Quality* 11(3):112-22, Fall 1996.

Jonathan Bogen, MSPH, MBA, CHE, is Founder of HealthCIO.com (www.healthcio.com), an on-line portal for medical information technology in Duxbury, Massachusetts.

CHAPTER 4

Use and Misuse of Physician Profiles
by Joseph A. Berry, MD, MBA

*T*o describe the health care environment today, one could easily apply the term chaotic, although complex may be more appropriate. There is rapid expansion of knowledge in medical science, which, in turn, has spawned a seemingly haphazard development of technologies in search of a cause. There are disconnected, inefficient, and disparate microsystems of health care delivery, and there are shifts in the global disease burden with the relatively recent emergence of deadly[1] infectious agents. These three factors alone lead to unpredictable patterns of care, unpredictable demands for services, less than optimal outcomes for the population in general, and uncontrolled costs. In this context, then, mechanisms that support and enable more rational demands for service and that allow us to understand the system of care delivery that leads increasingly to better outcomes for each health care dollar spent are desirable.

There are essentially three uses for physician profiles:

- Performance improvement.

- Physician selection.

- Discovery of relationships between processes and health care outcomes.

Together, these uses serve as a collective mechanism for attempting to bring some order out of chaos and some coherence to the complexity.

Historically, the subject of physician profiles has been the pattern of professional behavior reflected by utilization of resources, compliance with evidenced-based guidelines, clinical effectiveness, operational efficiency, service availability, practice styles, medical outcomes, billing practices, and costs. The inherent assumption is that, by profiling physicians and giving them feedback about their performance, a reduction in unexplained variation and a change in the professional behavior pattern toward some ideal state will occur over time. There are instances, however, in which the response of a physician to a profile needs to be more immediate and more predictable than what may arise from just a review of comparative feedback reports. In such instances when there is potential harm to individuals or to institutions, financial penalties may become the drivers of behavioral change in conjunction with profiles.

The major sources for performance improvement profiles are:

- Group practices with genuine concerns for improving the quality of care among members of the group.

- Capitated specialty groups that benefit by being more efficient and more effective in deploying appropriate resources.

- Federal and state agencies interested in ensuring adherence to regulations.

- Hospitals that need the close cooperation of physicians to exist.

- Managed care and other health care organizations that have a responsibility to make health care more affordable for more people.

- Teaching institutions that need to understand where best to place their emphasis in residency and community programs.

For specific examples of profiles tailored to modify professional behavior patterns, one can turn to the medical literature and to actual reports disseminated by organizations. An article in *Health Care Management Review* is illustrative. It reports a 23 percent reduction in ordering of ancillary services by physicians through the institution of a computerized audit and feedback program.[2] Balas *et al.*[3] conducted a meta-analysis of randomized clinical trials that tested the impact of physician profiling on the utilization of clinical procedures. The sources for their meta-analysis included health plans, medical centers, hospitals, and group practices. The physician profiling objectives ranged from influencing prescribing behavior, to test ordering practices, to the conduct of clinical screening. Heupler *et al.* reported how the results of quality of care profiles informed or directed specific performance improvement methods, such as education, clinical practice standardization, feedback and benchmarking, professional interaction, incentives, decision-support systems, and changes in administrative processes.[4] United HealthCare has conducted clinical profiles[5] to promote compliance with evidence-based guidelines and has provided physicians with not only the profiles but also a list of patients who may have eluded, for any number of reasons, the clinical intervention that the physicians intended to accomplish.

Selection

Whereas profiling to aid in the selection of physicians is not as studied and complicated an activity as profiling for performance improvement, it does constitute the more common use for profiling. Medical practice groups, IPAs, hospitals, managed care organizations, and universities profile physicians initially to determine whether or not a particular applicant for a position meets requirements and poses minimal risks to patients and liability to the group or institution. Credentialing, although not usually thought of as profiling, is an activity that assesses and compares physicians across multiple attributes and an activity that results in variable consequences, such as selection or deselection of physicians for medical staffs, group practices, or managed care networks. These attributes include but are not limited to specialty certification, prior work history, gaps in work history, residency program reputation and performance, procedures for which a physician has received formal training, committees on which a physician has participated, leadership roles in the medical community, contributions to medical studies, presentations, extent of continuing medical education and degree of continued exposure to academic medicine, hospital affiliations, liability history, and official sanctions. During reappointment cycles, additional attributes against which physicians are compared include complication rates for procedures, number of specific procedures performed per year, procedures or services per patient, percentage of compliance with well-established guidelines, and affordability.

Other sources of physician profiles for the purpose of aiding in the selection (or deselection) of physicians are state and federal agencies and proprietary consumer organizations. Profiling to confirm suspicions or complaints of abusive prescribing patterns has been part of the armamentarium of state agencies for years. These profiles increasingly form the basis of decisions to revoke or restrict physician licenses to the extent that they can help differentiate *appropriately* high narcotic prescribing patterns from *inappropriately* high prescribing patterns.[6] A more recent phenomenon that has evolved from state legislation is the publishing of physician profiles on the Internet. Massachusetts, for example, has led the way in providing health care consumers with physician profiles. The first section of the state's profile report provides general information about the physician, such as whether or not the physician is accepting new patients, the insurance plans accepted by the physician, hospital affiliations, and primary work setting. Section II covers education and training, while Section III specifies the area of specialty certification. Sections IV and V are the last of the self-reported areas of the profile and are used to highlight honors, awards, and professional publications. Sections VI and VII provide information about malpractice experience and disciplinary action. Both of these areas also have explanatory statements to help consumers put the negative information into some perspective.

Physician profiles generated at the federal level are linked to the sanctioning of physicians for billing abuse and fraud. Physicians with abusive billing practices are denied participation in federal programs. The following case histories are illustrative of physician profiles that have evolved with advances in artificial intelligence and that enable the culling out, from massive groupings of data, outlier physicians engaged in fraudulent practices.

CASE #1[7]
Billing Pattern
Codes Routinely Billed

Code	Procedure
G0001	Venipuncture
J1080	Injection of Testosterone Cypionate
54235	Injection of Corpora cavernosa
54240, 54250	Male Diagnostic Tests
81002	Chemstrip
82270	Fecal Occult Blood
95925	Doppler blood flow
99070	Office Visit to determine medication
99205	Comprehensive physical
99213	Exam second visit

Site of Care
Multiple states on the same dates.

Physician of Record
Although services were performed by locum tenens physicians and medical technologists, the "owning" physician was listed as the performing physician (the Q6 modifier was not employed as required).

CASE #2[8]
Billing Pattern
Codes Routinely Billed

Code	Procedure
95900	Nerve conduction; motor, each nerve
95904	Nerve conduction; sensory, each nerve
95925	Somatosensory testing, one or more nerves
93268	Patient demand single or multiple event recording
99203	Outpatient visit, new; detailed, low complexity
93930	Duplex scan of upper extremity arteries; bilateral
95935	"H" reflex test
99244	OV, new; comprehensive, moderate complexity

Site of Care
Four group practices in a large metropolitan area.

Physician of Record
General practitioners and family practitioners

■ Procedure codes 95900, 95904, 95925 are tests normally ordered by neurologists and rheumatologists. Orthopedic surgeons and doctors of internal medicine will also order these tests.

■ Procedure code 93268 represents a test normally ordered by cardiologists. Results are reviewed by a physician.

Physician profiling by state and federal agencies around patterns of resource utilization does not have as its objective the selection and deselection of physicians. If anything, these agencies serve as deterrents to health care organizations who may want to use profiling for this purpose. Legislation in the state of Rhode Island, for example, restrains a managed care organization from terminating a physician who does not practice cost effectively in the eyes of the MCO. If the determination is based on profiles, the organization must support its decision by demonstrating that adjustments were made in the profiles for severity of illness. Recent federal legislation impedes the termination of physicians from participation in the Medicare program on the basis of utilization profiles alone.

Before leaving selection as one of the uses for profiling, a reference about the emergence of proprietary consumer organizations is in order. In much the same fashion as pharmaceutical companies embracing the concept of disease management at the end of the eighties, marketing agencies are now picking up on the demand from the health care consumer for more information to aid them in the selection of physicians. One such company is called The Internet Directories.[9] The directory alleges the ability to provide consumers with information about physicians (and others) that will assist them in their selection. The following description is taken from its Web site:

"The Internet Directories is a corporation whose goal is to work with perspective advertising clients to give them tools tailored to their particular business such that these tools maximize the effectiveness of their advertising dollar.

"There are several ways that we seek to accomplish this goal. We have organized our directory such that it is very easy for a prospective user to obtain information on services, professions, and consumer goods on an industry or regional specific basis. As you browse our site you will note the ease at which a user is able to move from page to page and from state to state and gather information on the various goods and services offered and available within our many sub-directories."

As a health care directory, the site at this time lacks sufficient information on which a consumer can make decisions, but the potential is significant. Another well-publicized resource for consumer information about physicians in the form of profiles is Best Doctors. This company conducts a specialized consumer search. As its promotional material states, "Depending on the information available, the Care Consultant can determine not only the appropriate general area of expertise, but also the appropriate specialty (from 43 medical specialties), the appropriate subspecialty (from over 450 in the database), and, in some cases, the appropriate 'sub-subspecialty' (the individual doctor's special area of interest, experience, and/or research)." It is able to make this claim based on the array of attributes it maintains in its database on physicians across the country.

What the profiles of these two companies lack in validity, they make up for in meeting consumers' need for more information about their physicians than is generally available. There is currently no vehicle available, however, that has comprehensive and validated information that will satisfy the majority of instances in which a patient or family member is looking for an ideal match in terms of expertise, accessibility, availability, and style. Such sites, however, are beginning to emerge from health care organizations.

Discovery

The third use for physician profiling is in studying aspects of health care delivery or, more specifically, in discovering relationships between patterns of care and costs or between patterns of care and clinical outcomes. The first example of this use of profiling is a Medicaid study[10] that examines the relationship between cost performance and clinical performance among profiled physicians. In this study, it becomes apparent that a large number of physicians are misclassified regarding cost performance and, furthermore, that there is not a consistent association between cost performance and clinical performance (under the established parameters and study design). The objective of profiling in this situation is profiling itself, and the ability of this tool to illuminate the link between medical costs and performance.

A study on profiling by the University of Pittsburgh[11] offers a second example. The intent of this study is to understand the response of physicians to length-of-stay profiling. Its conclusion is that profiling does persuade physicians to reduce their patients' lengths of stay to the desired benchmark levels. It also raises a question for further discovery, " Why does profiling on the utilization of resources work well in some settings and not in others, for some resources and not others?"[12] These questions expose additional opportunities for discovering factors that may heighten one's ability to improve outcomes in a way that's affordable for everyone.

The last example is provided by a profiling project sponsored by the Robert Wood Johnson Foundation. This project is currently being conducted by an arm of the Medical Group Management Association. In this project, they have been able to demonstrate an ability to integrate information relating to physician work activity, as measured by Relative Value Units (RVUs), with practice and physician demographic information. The expectation is that their amassed database can be tapped into by others to study further the power and potential of physician profiling.

This use for profiling is no less prominent or important than the other two, and it is distinguished by its wider audience of end users. Organizations that develop this type of physician profiling include hospitals; group practices; pharmaceutical companies; disease management companies; universities; managed care organizations; foundations; and, to a diminishing extent, business coalitions.

Misuse of Profiling

Physician profiles are designed to promote some type of action-improve performance, differentiate and select "performers," inform policy, or understand processes. The resulting actions bring about unintended consequences if any of the following sins are committed:

- Profiling is considered a primary instrument of decision making rather than an adjunct to decision making.

- Physicians are not informed in advance of the assessment criteria or of the consequences of "outlier" performance.

- There is an absence of full disclosure regarding the methodology employed.

- The guidelines upon which the profile is based are invalid.

- There are flaws in the data input process.

- There is a failure to address the issue of case mix.

- The conclusions are based on small sample sizes or chance occurrences.[13]

In Case #2 above, the pattern of billing alone would have been insufficient information upon which to terminate the four physician groups from the program. The additional information that was obtained was that these groups hired marketing representatives to solicit patients 65 years old and older who had medical insurance. They enticed them through telemarketing, advertisements, church events, and random encounters in parks. The patients were told that the services were free and that they would be provided with transportation, meals, vitamins, etc. Once the groups obtained the patient's Medicare number, they billed Medicare for the procedures listed in the case example, whereas, in most cases, the services they received were limited to blood pressures checks and routine ECGs. The profiles in this situation served as an alert to fraudulent behavior.

Most profiles are derived from claims databases. While claims contain important information about care, they omit information that may be of equal or greater importance, such as results of tests, functional status of the patient, special physician training, competence of other physicians who managed the care of the patient, the fraction of the physician's practice devoted to procedures, and so on. The list of key variables, both dependent and independent, may be extensive; so that, even if the variables were available in one database, the challenge of coming to a rational conclusion can be great. The major sin to avoid among all of the seven is the third. There must be full disclosure of methodology to be fair to the physicians profiled and to be beneficial to the people who want the information.

Conclusion

In an excellent article about the ethical issues surrounding profiling and performance measures, Povar[14] writes that one of the justifications for these tools is "a health care professional's commitment to doing good" and knowing whether or not he or she is "doing good." He goes on to say that a "second reason is that we have a problem of the just allocation of scarce resources. If our practices are not efficient or parsimonious, we are essentially robbing the society of resources it needs to apply to other goods that it values. Indeed, clinicians may be among those who most appreciate the extent to which these other goods, such as housing, adequate nutrition, and education, have a great impact on health outcome indices."

What must be kept in the forefront of physician profiling, therefore, are the ultimate objectives of continually changing medical practice for the better and improving outcomes.

References and Footnotes

1. "Like the brief doomed flare of exploding suns that register dimly on blind men's eyes, the beginning of the horror passed almost unnoticed; in the shriek of what followed, in fact, was forgotten and perhaps not connected to the horror at all."—*The Exorcist*, by William Peter Blatty, 1971.

2. Braham, R., and Ruchlin, H. "Physician Practice Profiles: A Case Study of the Use of Audit and Feedback in an Ambulatory Care Group Practice." *Health Care Management Review* 12(3):11-6, Summer 1987.

3. Balas, E., and others. "Effect of Physician Profiling on Utilization." *Journal of General Internal Medicine* 11(10):584-90, Oct. 1996.

4. Heupler, F., and others. "Guidelines for Internal Peer Review in the Cardiac Catheterization Laboratory." *Catheterization and Cardiovascular Diagnosis* 40(1):21-32, Jan. 1997.

5. Newcomer, L. "Physician, Measure Thyself." *Health Affairs* 17(4):32-5, July-Aug. 1998.

6. Virginia Board of Medicine revoked a Washington, D.C., physician's license for overprescribing narcotics to chronic pain patients. This case gained national notoriety when presented on the CBS-TV news show "60 Minutes."

7. HCFA RMFA 9613, Nov. 14, 1996.

8. HCFA RMFA 9608, Oct. 23, 1996.

9. http://www.theinternetdirectories.com/

10. Powe, N., and others. "Systemwide Performance in a Medicaid Program: Profiling the Care of Patients with Chronic Illnesses." *Medical Care* 34(8):798-810, Aug. 1996.

11. Evans, J., and others. Physician Response to Length of Stay Profiling." *Medical Care* 33(11):1106-19, Nov. 1995.

12. Balas, A., *et al.*, *op. cit.* In the meta-analysis, profiling had a minimal effect on the utilization of procedures. None of the studies looked at utilization of hospital days.

13. Brand, D., and others. "Data Needs of Profiling Systems." In Physician *Payment Review Commission Conference on Profiling*, No. 92-2. Washington, D.C.: Physician Payment Review Commission, 1992, pp. 20-45.

14. Povar, G. "Profiling and Performance Measures. What Are the Ethical Issues." *Medical Care* 33(1, Suppl.):JS60-8, Jan. 1995.

Joseph A. Berry, MD, MBA, is National Medical Director, United HealthCare, Edina, Minnesota.

CHAPTER 5

The Process of Physician Profiling
by John B. Coombs, MD, and
Margaret H. Gilshannon, MHA

Case Scenarios in Physician Profiling
Scenario A

Y ou are the medical director of a large multispecialty clinic. The medical executive of the area's largest health plan has just called you to let you know that, unless you can provide outcomes data to justify your costs, your contract will not be renewed. The health plan is looking to cut costs, and if you can't demonstrate the quality and cost-effectiveness of your physicians, you'll lose your biggest contract.

You ask the quality improvement director to tell you what kind of inpatient and outpatient physician- and department-specific data he can give you as quickly as possible. You need to present the news to your physicians at the upcoming monthly medical staff meeting. You need to convince them that profiling their practices is the only way to begin to demonstrate the clinic's quality and outcomes to the health plan. And you need to tell them that, if the profiles don't show favorable results, physicians will need to make changes in their practice patterns.

What approach might you take (both short and long term) to:

■ *Get your physicians to "buy in" to the profiling process?*

■ *Integrate the physician profiling process into your ongoing quality improvement efforts?*

■ *Address physicians or groups of physicians who may look "worse" than others in the profile?*

■ *Work with management to address health plan concerns that may arise from the data?*

Scenario B

You are the vice president for medical affairs of a community hospital, and the largest health plan you contract with has just mailed to you and to the physicians on your medical staff the physicians' annual practice profiles. The profiles include the following measures: average length of stay per DRG, cost per DRG, pharmacy utilization, laboratory and radiology utilization, readmission rates, and patient satisfaction scores.

You have several concerns. Are these data accurate-how did the health plan collect the data, and did your physicians and staff report accurately? Do the data match your data-are you and the health plan measuring indicators in the same way; if not, do you agree with the way in which they are measuring? Are the data relevant-do they really measure what they claim to measure, and are the measures clinically meaningful? Have the data been case-mix adjusted? If so, is the method of severity adjustment the same method used for your data?

Scenario C

You are the medical director of a large health plan and are embarking on a process to profile the practices of physicians with whom you contract. You would like to use these profiles to help get some of your most costly physician groups in line with cost and utilization patterns of your average physician group. You need to figure out what data you will collect and what measures you will report in your profiles. You also need to determine how to present the data to help create incentives for providers to achieve certain benchmarks. Your goal is to link the profiles with physicians' production and to demonstrate to some of your high-cost physician groups that good outcomes can be achieved with a different approach to patient management.

What approach should you take in:

■ *Determining which indicators are best suited to your objective?*

■ *Determining the benchmarks you want to use to establish incentives for your providers?*

■ *Presenting the profiles to meet your desired goals?*

Embarking on the Profiling Process

Each of these scenarios illustrates a set of common principles that characterize contemporary medical management. First, outcomes data play an increasingly important role in shaping medical practice as we move from implicit to explicit means of measuring utilization and quality. Second, efforts to remove unexplained (or unnecessary) variation have become the central means of recognizing improved value in health care delivery. Third, involvement of physicians, along with hospitals, group practices, and payers, is essential to creating change in the content and the pattern of care delivery and to moving quality and cost toward greater value within the delivery system.

In addition, the move from an implicitly to an explicitly defined method of delivering health care has added momentum to the emergence of evidence-based medicine (EBM). EBM is the incorporation of four components into an explicitly defined system of care delivery:

■ Scientific evidence appraisal.

■ Clearly defined processes of care delivery (such as care maps, critical paths and disease management).

■ Decision-making support.

■ Outcomes measurement.

The goal in explicitly defining each component within this evidence-based system is to eliminate unnecessary variation and provide optimal value and outcome for the patient.

Physician practice profiling provides a means by which one can simultaneously present data which reflect individual physician practice characteristics, demonstrate variation among providers, and create a means by which physicians can participate in improving practice patterns.

Profiling can be an important tool in facilitating provider feedback, communication, and defining actionable items upon which EBM can be continuously modified. Essential to the success of this effort is a careful process that introduces and develops consensus around intent, as well as discusses a number of issues critical to meaningful participation of physicians. This chapter explores the essential elements of a successful process for implementation and ongoing support of physician profiling.

Key Process Steps

Lasker *et al.*[1] point out that "the ultimate objective of profiling is to change medical practice for the better" and that "providers will probably be reluctant to change their behavior unless a particular profile convinces them that action is warranted."[2] Other authors have written about the essential elements in the process of establishing a profiling system[3]. First and foremost, profiles must lead to or be part of an overall strategy to support change. This could include identification of a key clinical process of care that can be modified using the technique of continuous quality improvement (CQI)[4]. In an inpatient setting, this could include introduction or modification of a care map or a critical pathway. Likewise, in an ambulatory setting, profiling might set the scene and motivate practitioners to establish and implement a disease management process for a chronic medical problem such as diabetes or hypertension. Regardless, profiling data must lead to a process by which physician interest and efforts to change can be focused and operationalized. The process leading to collection, analysis, and distribution of profiles should contain, at a minimum, the following steps:

1. Discuss the rationale for profiling with physicians who will be involved-why profile?

2. Support the rationale by defining for physicians and the institution (hospital, practice, payer, etc.) the benefits of creating the profiled information.

3. Establish which data will be used and what specific data elements are best suited for the intended purpose of the profile.

4. Develop policy about who will have access to the profiled information and the rules that will govern confidentiality and appropriate use of the data.

5. Discuss accuracy along with strengths and weaknesses of the profiled information.

6. Address concerns that might exist within the group regarding small numbers, case mix (severity), etc.

7. Define the process of change that might be used to create an actionable outcome from the available profiles.

8. Measure outcomes from changes that are made as a result of the profiles-share outcomes information and profiles that are developed after changes are implemented.

Throughout the process, it is critical that the process director remain flexible and open while reminding the group of what consensus objectives and decisions have already been made. The director's patience and willingness to listen are essential elements.

Why Profile?

Many different applications of profiled information can prove valuable to practicing physicians. As classically trained scientists, all physicians respond to data and information and generally are aware of the characteristics of good data and of statistical and epidemiological methods. Therefore, creating timely information about an ongoing clinical problem and collecting, organizing, and feeding back information in a "user-friendly" fashion promote constructive action. In different settings, the rationale for profiling might differ dramatically, but, beyond creating information feedback, profiling can also accomplish or support the following goals:

1. Support an institution's quality assessment and assurance program with performance-based credentialing and tracking of key clinical indicators by provider.

2. Monitor indicators that either reflect adverse events or record their occurrence within a risk management program.

3. Support process change (CQI, pathway development, disease management).

4. Create a forum for providers to discuss unexplained variation and set direction for enhancing value and reducing variation.

5. Allow providers to respond to externally generated data that threaten market position, quality reputation, and purchaser perception.

6. Enhance payer value and reduce inappropriate care and costs.

7. Assess provider performance, routinely, if desired.

8. Enable organizations interested in better managing care to select the most efficient providers.

The rationale for profiling information is often influenced by the motivation of provider groups or payers when they recognize the need to begin a process of change. Factors that might heighten motivation include a sentinel event (e.g., death of an asthmatic in the clinic), high cost (for either providers at risk or payers), hassle and confusion in providing care, or establishment of an external benchmark in a highly competitive environment. All of these factors can heighten the interest and "buy in" of key participants and should be recognized as opportunities upon which to build.

Closely related to motivation is the issue of defining benefits for participants in a process of change. A multitude of factors must be considered and brought before any group engaged in the developmental phase of the change process. Efficiency and providing "best practice" (in a quality sense), while reducing cost and increasing profitability, all need to be considered and defined for the specific project being undertaken. Frequently, greater efficiency of care leads to heightened productivity on the part of the participating provider, as well as greater derived satisfaction from the practice of medicine. In a time of increasing demands on the provider to do more with less, enhancing productivity and individual satisfaction can be a godsend.

Which Data?

Selecting the proper data elements, on the basis of availability, is critical to the success of any effective profiling process. While this step is discussed in greater detail below, failure to recognize the shortcomings of available data can create chaos in the group process to establish profiling and support change. Small numbers, untrimmed data containing outliers, lack of severity adjustment, or aggregation of dissimilar data all can spell disaster in mounting a successful profiling effort. While assembled data may not allow for "pure science," recognizing the weaknesses of a given data set might allow its use in management guidance supporting the process of "educated change." In its purest sense, this is often a difficult concept for physicians to accept and allows those who might not fully support constructive change to undermine the process.

Elements of Success

Whether the focus of the profiling exercise is on demonstrating variation, quantifying and tracking performance, or improving quality by implementing a clearly defined process of care, several elements of success associated with the profiling process are apparent. First, the focus of profiles must not be only on outcomes measures but also on indicators that reflect how well the defined process of care is working. Second, confidential feedback of physician-specific data is essential to maintain physician trust while clearly keeping the focus on change for the better. Third, the presence of a physician champion who commands the respect of other physicians and is able to work as an opinion leader and mentor for the group enhances the chances of success. Investing time and training in such a potential champion is worth the resources. Fourth, expect slow, incremental progress in developing the process that supports profiling. Allow plenty of time for the physician group to understand the strengths and the weaknesses of the data and to create policy around how to use and apply the data. Finally, be sure to clearly define the potential derived benefit from profiling data, the information that can be gained from it and the process of change that it will support. Efficiency of care and enhanced quality of care and outcomes (including minimizing adverse events) that can evolve from the process will provide ample benefit and satisfaction to participating physicians when carefully defined early in the process.

Combining Intent, Content, and Format

Depending on the objective of the process and the intention of the profiling organization, content, focus, and format may differ dramatically. Payers may want to provide coded, confidential feedback on utilization of resources to providers within their health plan to periodically inform them of their utilization relative to other physicians in the plan. An example of this form of feedback is contained in figure 1, below, which profiles either coded interests or family physicians, utilization of consultative specialty care measured in dollars spent per member per month ($/MM) as well as $/MM spent on primary care visits. Information is easy to read and interpret. Care is taken to maintain the anonymity of providers. The profile shows a plan average that indicates that most of the physicians profiled are above the average spent per member month across the plan. Profiles such as these from payers create their own "sentinel effect" among providers, encouraging them to ask themselves why their personal profile is above or below the average. Likewise, if a physician is in an extreme position compared to other providers, corrective evaluation and action can occur. Periodically publishing the profile allows individual physicians to track their performance over time.

In another example taken from a hospital setting, providers of transurethral resection of the prostate (TURP) are profiled using length of hospital stay and

FIGURE 1.

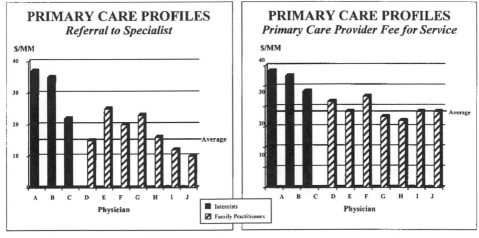

Payer profile of primary care physician utilization of specialty care recorded in dollars per member month ($/MM) and $/MM expended on primary care services in discounted fee-for-service HMO.

FIGURE 2.

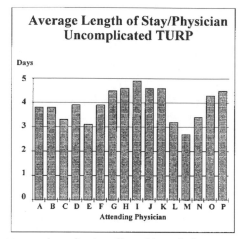

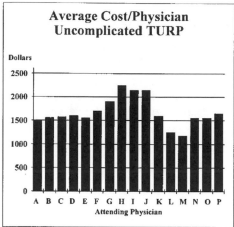

Hospital medical staff profiles of physician practice pattern characteristics for a surgical procedure.

average cost for individual coded physicians (figure 2, above). The absence of benchmarks, averages, or any form of severity adjustment limits how this information can be applied.

During the process of establishing a physician group, discussion of the data presents the opportunity to demonstrate variation and to improve the quality and the accuracy of the data by asking for physician input. These profiles can then be used to engage physicians in developing a care map for postoperative care or in participating in a quality improvement exercise aimed at increasing hospital efficiency and patient satisfaction. Whereas the payer profiling process is primarily aimed at performance feedback and self-directed change as a result of sentinel effect, the profiles in figure 2 were developed to support the formation of a group of physicians to work on process refinement within a hospital setting. These examples represent similar formats with different purposes defined by the process of development and by the objectives of the initiator.

A final example of how intent, content, and format can come together is provided in figure 3, page 69. In this example, an employer-purchasers association has profiled, by physician group, hospital charges and length of hospital stay incurred during C-section. Physicians may or may not have been involved in the development of this profile. Rather, like the payer example above, the intent of the profile is to get the attention of the physicians and encourage improvement in a competitive marketplace. This example introduces several formatting nuances. First, the data are presented in a bi-dimensional format, allowing two variables to be seen simultaneously. Second, the names of the physician groups

FIGURE 3.

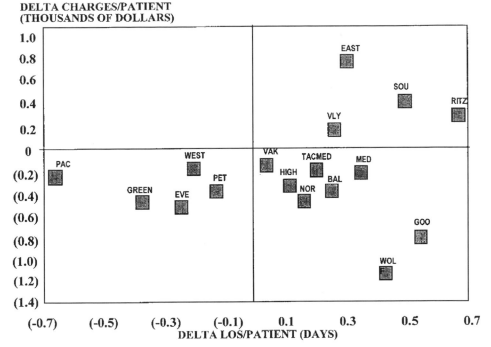

Physician group practices: comparison of hospital length of stay and patient charges for patients undergoing Caesarean section (without comorbidity).

are clearly displayed, adding the likelihood of threat to the data presentation and potentially creating motivation. This approach might also spawn animosity such that a constructive call to action may quickly become a defensive "call to arms." By formatting data on C-section rates, the profiler hopes providers will respond to an opportunity for improvement, in this case, excessive hospital cost and length of stay.

As the previous examples have illustrated, the method of communicating information is critical to the success of a physician profiling process. In general, to keep focus on the objectives of the profiling process, it's important to avoid categorizing providers and data as either "good" or "bad." The profiling process is intended to look for unexplained variation among providers and for areas of deviation from a standard or a guideline. Therefore, the communication process should focus on education for improvement rather than single out "poor" performers.[4]

The objective for profiling, whether for a hospital, a health plan, or a provider group, may vary. How profiles are presented and communicated will affect your ability to achieve the goals of the profiling process. For example, if you represent a health plan and your main objective is to reduce costs, you will be most interested in presenting the cost and the utilization profiles of your providers and in comparing them to some standard or example of best practice. Or your objectives may be to reduce pharmacy costs, and you may want to limit your focus, for example, to pharmacy utilization patterns. To illustrate, in table 1, below, a profile of a hospital's cardiologists includes admissions and charge data to determine a physician inpatient resource score (PIRS), which is compared to peer groups across the state. The percentile rankings are helpful in presenting the comparison groups against whom a physician is benchmarked. These comparison groups could be, as they are in this example, peer group physicians at the same hospital, peer group physicians practicing in the local area, peer group physicians practicing in the broader region, and all peer group physicians in the state.

TABLE 1. PHYSICIAN CHARGE AND ADMISSION DATA[4]

Physician	PIRS	Admissions	Case Mix	Charge Index	Per Day Index
A	1%	28	0.97	0.89	0.71
B	4%	100	1.17	0.93	0.99
C	7%	39	0.95	0.96	0.74
D	9%	87	1.01	1.06	1.00
E	20%	38	1.20	1.15	1.01
F	23%	26	0.97	0.99	0.93
G	38%	83	0.97	1.16	1.09
H	77%	62	1.04	1.12	1.10
I	85%	50	0.79	1.29	1.25
J	89%	36	0.94	1.15	1.21
K	90%	93	0.98	1.25	1.12
L	95%	32	0.87	1.18	1.31
M	97%	27	0.75	1.24	1.25
N	98%	50	0.96	1.23	1.07

*PIRS (Physician Inpatient Resource Scores) represent percentile ranking within peer group across the state. High scores suggest higher resource use. In addition, Index = actual/expected (case mix and severity-adjusted).

In another example from the same hospital, orthopedic surgeons' charge and length-of-stay indexes are benchmarked on a severity and case-mix adjusted basis (figure 4, page 71). Each "bubble" represents an individual physician, and the bubble size corresponds to the relative number of discharges, which also adds the element of volume or productivity. This illustration demonstrates the correlation between length of stay and charge indexes in a visually compelling fashion. With minimal interpretation, the graphical representation of data conveys the relationship between length of stay and charges.

FIGURE 4. Profile of a hospital's orthopedic surgeon's LOS index versus charge index.[4]

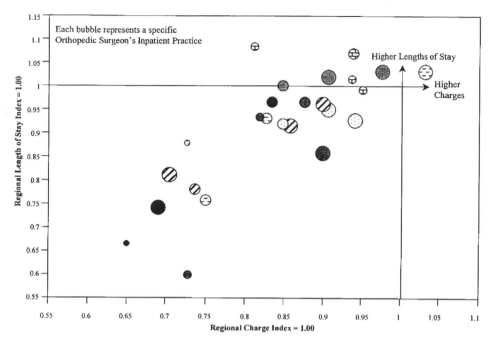

An effective means of comparing cost, utilization, process, and outcome data is through what are sometimes referred to as "dashboard indicator reports." These reports lay out, in plain view, a series of measures or indicators of care processes and outcomes. Setting various indicators of quality, service, and cost of a care process alongside one another can give a broad overview of an individual physician's practice, or they can be aggregated to illustrate a department, clinic, or hospital's overall profile. Report cards such as these are another method of providing comparable performance information that can be tracked and trended over time.

In table 2, page 72, indicators of quality, service, and utilization are profiled for a managed care setting. A given practice or group is compared to the health plan's benchmark. Quality is measured through indicators of member satisfaction, chart reviews, member transfer rates, and adherence to the managed care philosophy. Overall service or comprehensiveness of care is measured through such indicators as number of scheduled office hours, internal practice coverage, patient management services, and practice growth. Finally, indicators of utilization in this profile include a measure of practices' use of hospital services, specialty services, and emergency department services. In a simple-to-follow format, this quality report card illustrates the measures that are important to this health plan and how a given

TABLE 2. Profile of quality, services and utilization indicators in a managed care setting used for the purpose of calculating financial reimbursement.[5]

Components of quality factor	Highest possible scores or range (%)	Scores for ABC Practice
Quality review (36% or total)		
Member satisfaction survey results	-0.75 to 3.00	2.00
Focused chart review findings	-0.75 to 3.00	0.75
Member transfer rate	-0.75 to 1.50	0.50
Adherence to managed care philosophy	-0.75 to 3.00	1.00
Total for quality review	**-3.00 to 10.50**	**4.25**
Comprehensive Care (47% of total)		
Membership size (1 for 250 members per doctor; 0.5 for each additional 250)	2.00	1.00
Scheduled office hours (0.5 for 50 hours/week; 0.5 for each additional 10 hours/week)	1.50	0.50
Office procedures offered (1 for each; max of 3)	3.00	1.00
Program education courses completed (0.5 for each course)	2.00	0.50
Internal practice coverage (if physicians cover for one another)	1.00	1.00
Catastrophic care (if practice managers difficult cases)	1.50	1.50
Patient management (if practice works with HMO's services)	1.00	1.00
Computer link to network (if practice is linked)	1.0	1.00
Total for comprehensive care	**14.00**	**8.50**
Utilization (17% of total)		
Hospital services	-0.80 to 1.80	0.80
Specialty services	-0.80 to 1.80	0.40
Emergency department services	-0.80 to 1.40	0.60
Total for utilization	**-2.40 to 5.00**	**1.80**
Total quality factor	**29.50**	**14.55**

practice compares to the health plan's benchmark or ideal practice in an attempt to align physician's financial incentives with what the plan considers optimal practice behavior.

Finding the Data

Information, appropriately profiled and created from refinement of available data, provides the power to promote change and improvement in both processes of care and outcomes. Critical to acceptance of profiled information is an understanding of where it came from and its accuracy. As classically trained scientists, physicians know that incorrect data will lead to conclusions without foundation. As a consequence, bad data will lead to the loss of participant trust and to failure to create positive and enduring change.

Two areas provide fertile ground when looking for critical data that reflect processes underpinning care and outcomes. First are components that make for value in health care: appropriateness, quality of care, quality of service, and cost. Second, and somewhat overlapping, are the four areas contained in outcomes measurement: quality indicators, patient and provider satisfaction, functional status, and cost-related indicators. These two general areas, plus indicators that reflect the process of care delivery (such as training in medication distribution or availability of physical therapy after joint replacement), provide excellent content for profiles that can be used in quality improvement or performance measurement.

There is increased attention on outcome measures by the Joint Commission on Accreditation of Healthcare Organizations (JCAHO) and the National Committee on Quality Assurance (NCQA). JCAHO's IM System and closely associated data-driven ORYX accrediting system provide a variety of quality indicators now being kept by hospitals and hospital systems (www.jcaho.org). NCQA, with the development of the Health Plan Employer Data Information System (HEDIS), provides a full complement of data elements from health plans and aggregates reporting of quality indicators by health plans in its publicly available Quality Compass (www.ncqa.com). In addition, patient and provider satisfaction surveys are now conducted by most health care organizations and health plans, making this a good source of profilable information.

As noted by Brand *et al.*,[6] sources of data must be accurate, representative (unbiased), accessible (particularly enhanced when electronically collected at the time of service without the need for separate entry), and relevant to the task at hand.

To date, administrative data sets (such as claims data and charge data from providers) have been an important source of information. Many excellent critiques of these sources of data are available in the literature.[6-8] Claims data are attractive because they are electronically stored and share many common characteristics across different payers. In addition, numbers are large, which reduces bias. Also, claims data frequently contain information on individuals over time and in a variety of settings. Limitations exist, in that information is frequently most complete in the hospital setting and less so in ambulatory points of services. Gaps in care or other technical issues surrounding filing of claims often exist. A variety of other drawbacks exist and are either more completely reviewed below or are beyond the scope and focus of this discussion.

Other Data Considerations

Because of the importance of accuracy and the need to reduce as much as possible any bias from information used in profiling, a number of other factors need to be considered. These include small numbers, case-mix or severity adjustment, outliers (whether to trim and how), validity of aggregating data (pooling data across clinics or physicians), and benchmarks. Several of these areas deserve additional comment.

Small Numbers

When working on processes of care within practices or institutions, small numbers are often difficult to avoid. The presence of small numbers may significantly limit conclusions from a study for which all that exists is a limited sample. However, recognizing and acknowledging this fact is often half the battle.

Case Mix/Severity of Illness

Adjusting data for case mix or severity of illness is a critical consideration, especially when profiling individual physicians. When confronted with unfavorable variation, a physician might reply, "But my patients are sicker." Many reviews have been written on this topic both in the inpatient setting[9,10] and the ambulatory setting.[11-17] Suffice it to say that no existing system or approach provides the entire answer and is applicable to all situations. However, the opportunity exists to substantially improve the representative nature of data by applying some form of case mix or severity adjustment.

Briefly summarizing available severity adjustment systems, table 3, page 75, examines inpatient systems and compares several shared variables, including the basis upon which severity is measured, data requirements, and the unit of classification.

Table 4, page 75, lists five systems for case-mix adjustment available for use in the ambulatory setting. Unlike most hospital data, which are available through automated retrieval, ambulatory data are most frequently found in paper charts or in gap-filled claims information. Consequently, universal application of ambulatory severity adjustment is behind that of hospital data sets.

TABLE 3. Risk Adjustment Systems Designed for Application in the Inpatient Setting

Severity Adjustment System	Basis of Severity	Applied to Whom	Unit of Classification	Data Source
All Patient Refined DRGS (APR DRGS)	Relative Hospital Charges • Comorbid • Conditions • Complications	All Inpatients	Disease and Patient	Discharge Abstract
Acute Physiology and Chronic Health Evaluation (APACHE II)	• ICU Oriented • Risk of Imminent Death	All ICU Patients	Patient	Medical Record
MEDISGROUPS	Clinical Status	All Inpatients	Patient	Medical Record
Computerized Severity Index (CSI)	• LOS Reflecting • Treatment Complexity	700 Diagnostic Categories	Disease and Patient	Medical Record
Disease Staging	Extent of Organ System Involvement	400 Diagnostic Categories	Disease	Medical Record

TABLE 4. Severity adjustment systems directed at the ambulatory setting[7,14]

Measure	Primary Purpose	Unit of Analysis	Inputs
Diagnosis Clusters	Measure Content of Care	Visit	Primary Diagnosis
Ambulatory Visit Groups (AVGs)	Define Products of Care	Visit	Primary Diagnosis Procedures Age & Sex Disposition
Ambulatory Patient Groups (APGs)	Medicare Reimbursement	Visit	Primary Diagnosis Procedures Age & Sex Disposition
Ambulatory Care Groups (ACGs)	Predict Resource Use Set Capitation Rates	One Year	All Diagnoses Age & Sex

In addition to the systems listed in table 4, severity adjustment using outpatient drug dispensing databases has also been researched and is currently being used in many settings, primarily in HMOs.[15] Within managed care organizations, the use of drug dispensing data for severity adjustment has been particularly useful, given that claims data are often not collected on physician visits.

Benchmarks

The limited availability of comparisons across providers, especially in highly competitive markets in which public databases are not mandated, has significantly hampered efforts at benchmarking. Likewise, beyond local markets, if a provider is not part of a larger regional or national system, benchmarks are difficult to obtain. Establishment of standardizing indicators such as JCAHO'S IM System and NCQA's HEDIS should lessen this problem over time. Similarly, groups such as the Center for Research in Ambulatory Health Care Administration (CRAHCA) have established efforts to create comparative ambulatory databases.[18] The absence of benchmarks or national standard data sets limits the overall measurement of quality and the ability of providers to establish minimum performance standards.

Finally, when thinking about strengths and weaknesses of a database, one must recognize the importance of statistical methods when evaluating data.

CQI, Evidence-Based Medicine, and Administrative Oversight

Integrating physician practicing profiling into an organization's quality improvement process is an important application of the valuable data obtained through profiling. More recently, physician profiling has become integral in the emergence of evidence-based medicine. Continuous quality improvement (CQI) takes traditional quality assurance a step further by presenting a method for assessing and managing performance indicators. The goal of the CQI process is to use knowledge (or evidence) for improvement. The plan-do-study-act (PDSA) cycle (figure 5, page 77) can be used as a framework for incorporating profiling into a CQI process. Profiling represents the "study" or "check" part of the cycle by providing feedback to physicians on the patterns of their practice.

In the first step, a process for improvement is identified (Plan). Process improvements are then made, and data are collected about those improvements (Do). In the third step, data are reviewed or profiled to check for improvement (Study). Based on conclusions drawn from the profiles, the improvement process continues (Act). In this illustration, the profile is a method of auditing a process and then feeding back the results of the audit into the process. The goal is always to study and act for education and

FIGURE 5. The "Plan, Do, Study, Act" Cycle as part of a CQI process.

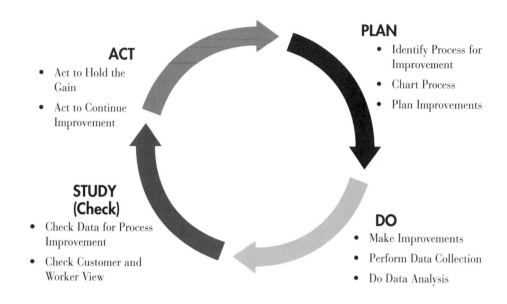

ACT
- Act to Hold the Gain
- Act to Continue Improvement

PLAN
- Identify Process for Improvement
- Chart Process
- Plan Improvements

STUDY (Check)
- Check Data for Process Improvement
- Check Customer and Worker View

DO
- Make Improvements
- Perform Data Collection
- Do Data Analysis

improvement and to continually take into account variations and changes that occur in various processes over time. In this way, a CQI process and the profiling process that feeds into it are never static, but are always encouraging learning and changing for improvement.

An organization employing EBM's methodologies is in many senses applying the principles of CQI to its clinical care delivery system. Profiles can be used effectively in developing evidence-based best practices. As the evidence-driven audit cycle illustrates (figure 6, page 78), critically appraised evidence is used to develop clinical practice guidelines for the treatment of a given population or disease. Performance against those guidelines is measured and incorporated into a physician practice profile. This profile is then used to identify unexplained practice variation and forms a basis upon which physicians can alter their practice patterns. This method for developing evidence-based best practices represents the use of clinical information in an audit/feedback loop very similar to the PDSA cycle.

In addition to clinical management of a care delivery system, physician practice profiling can also be used in the management and oversight of health care delivery. Physician profiles can be used in initial credentialing processes to determine if a new physician is appropriate for inclusion in a physician practice or health plan or on a hospital's medical staff. Following initial

FIGURE 6. The evidence-driven audit cycle.[19]

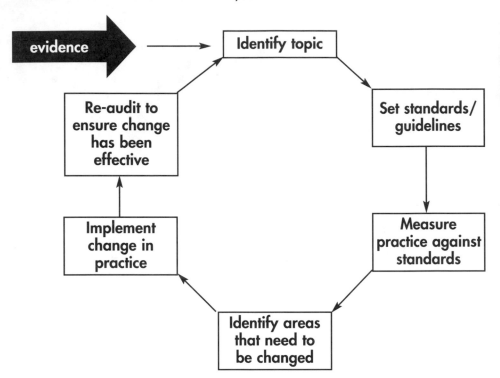

appointment, performance-based profiles can be used in a regular recredentialing process to assess and compare performance and to adjust referral patterns or reimbursement mechanisms. Profiles also provide information to an
organization's governing body. A simplified presentation of key quality indicators, especially when trended over time and combined with goals or benchmarks, can support the decision-making process of management and governance groups that may not be familiar with the clinical details of care delivery. In addition, processes can be profiled to support operational compliance
or to track progress by illustrating utilization and cost patterns that can
affect operational and strategic decision making. As when using profiles to
motivate physicians to change their practice patterns, the objectives of using
profiles in management and the setting of the organization can determine the
method and the format of communication. For example, the lay volunteer
board of a community hospital may look differently at profiles than the
financial oversight committee of a large health plan. Carefully thinking
through which data will be meaningful to the group, and how to most effectively present the data to achieve the intended objectives of the profiling
process, is critical to effective use of physician practice profiles.

TABLE 5. Approaches to changing physician practice patterns. Profiling can be used as a specific tool for communicating information in a variety of these examples.

Intervention	Intervention format
Education	
Continuing Medical Education	Didactic Educational Experiences
Individual and Small Group CME	Focused Tutorials
Opinion Leader	Respected Colleague "Coaching" [22,23]
Academic Detailing	Short, 1 to 1 Communication[24]
Patient Centered Strategies	Focused on Soliciting Patient Preferences[25]
Feedback	
Feedback with Audit	Performance Feedback Profiles

Process Participation

Critical Pathway/Care Map Development	Explicit Precess Definition[26]
Continuous Quality Improvement (CQI)	Remainders Presenting "Best Practice"
Clinical Decision Support	

Administrative
Formulary Development
　Required Consultation (Limited Credentialing)

Financial Incentives/Penalties[5]

Changing Physician Practice Patterns

For profiling to be an effective tool in promoting communication and change, it must be combined with a specific change strategy. In their 1993 article, Greco and Eisenberg[20] outline the five general strategies for changing physician practices: education, feedback, participation in processes of change, administrative intervention (regulation), and financial incentives or penalties.

Within these general categories, specific interventions have been devised and implemented. Table 5, above, outlines these approaches within the general categories. Under education, a variety of approaches may be used, depending on the change that is being considered. As an example, the use of academic detailing has been successfully applied when promoting the use of effective medications. Patient-centered strategies acknowledge the importance of offering patients informed choices at critical therapeutic intervention points, such as choosing a surgical approach versus watchful waiting versus a medical approach.

The scope of this chapter does not allow for a comprehensive discussion of each of these change strategies. However, physician profiling may apply to most of these approaches as a tool for communication and measurement of outcomes once an intervention has been put into place. As an example, introducing a practice profile that demonstrates specific physician data and variation among a group of physicians practicing in the locale will increase the degree of interest that might surround an educational program or intervention by an opinion leader. Experience tells us that physician profiling in this instance is most effective when the topic to be addressed has been identified by the targeted physician group as an area of interest or as a key quality concern. Likewise, in optimizing the change strategy, the use of current information and the production of timely feedback once the intervention has been put in place most often produce the best results. Davis[27] extensively explores these various approaches that promote change in behavior and provides an excellent summary of what is currently known about their effectiveness in specific settings. What is critical to our discussion here is that, within the process of developing a profiling system, one must recognize the importance of profiling as a means of communication that demonstrates actionable information and leads to an implementable plan for changing practice patterns and promoting improvement.

Concluding Remarks and Summary

This chapter has reviewed the eight essential steps to ensuring a successful profiling process:

1. **Tell the physicians why you're profiling.** Get their involvement and support at the beginning of the process. Take time to solicit their input on the "rules" that will apply to the profiling process. Clearly state your objectives and reiterate them frequently to maintain your focus.

2. **Define the benefits of creating the profiles.** Be clear in embarking on a profiling process on how the process and its outcomes will benefit physicians and the organization.

3. **Determine the best data for your intended purpose.** Don't use data just because they are available. Focus on your intended purpose, and, from the available data, select the elements that will directly assist you in meeting your objectives.

4. **Develop policies about access, use, and confidentiality.** Anticipate potential problems and address them in clear and well-understood policies on which physicians and managers agree.

5. **Discuss the accuracy, strengths, and weaknesses of the data.** Be open and honest with physicians and others about the potential limitations of the profiled information, while remaining focused on your objectives.

6. **Refine the data.** To enhance the credibility of the data and the process, develop procedures for adjusting and accounting for variation in data that are not related to physicians' practice behavior. Address concerns about small numbers, case mix, etc.

7. **Focus on actionable outcomes.** Direct the profiling process toward items that are actionable and that can lead to a process of change that will favorably influence outcomes. Focus on outcomes that physicians can "do something about," rather than on areas in which change would be complicated and difficult to achieve.

8. **Measures outcomes after change implementation.** Demonstrate improvements made after beginning the profiling process, and track these changes over time. Feedback is an essential element in supporting changes.

In reviewing the case scenarios at the beginning of this chapter, think about how these process steps can be applied in addressing the problem faced in each scenario.

While focusing on the essential process steps, it's important to avoid several potential pitfalls. First, beware of moving ahead too fast before achieving clarity on your goals and objectives, communicating effectively with your physicians, and ensuring that appropriate data are available. Second, throughout the process but especially when just beginning, carefully protect confidentiality. To ensure physician support of the process, issues around the protection of data need to be resolved up front. Third, the profiling process can fall apart if leadership does not acknowledge the potential shortfalls of the data and the process. It's important to admit that you may not have perfect data and to acknowledge where the weaknesses may lie and what will be done to address them. Be aware that physicians may be skeptical of the use of management data that can help guide a manager's actions but may not reflect "pure science."

Significant problems encountered in the profiling process can seriously undermine overall objectives. Nevertheless, profiling skeptics such as Kassirer encourage physicians to "be open-minded about the concept of practice profiles, engage actively in developing the methods to be used, help determine whether the effort and cost of refining them is worth it, and test them in the field. If it can be demonstrated that they reflect the nature and variety of a physician's patients, the process of care, and the outcomes of a physician's decisions, those who practice good medicine and do not exploit resources for personal gain should have nothing to fear."[28] American Medical News reported that the climate for profiling is changing, moving from "being perceived as an unnecessary evil to a necessary evil to, today, a necessary good"[29]. As physicians and organizations struggle to begin practice profiling efforts, outlining the process and its objectives remains critical to ensuring success in improving practice patterns to achieve better clinical outcomes.

References

1. Lasker, R., and others. "Realizing the Potential of Practice Pattern Profiling." *Inquiry* 29(3):287-97, Fall 1992.

2. Garnick, D., and others. "Focus on Quality: Profiling Physicians' Practice Patterns." *Journal of Ambulatory Care Management* 17(3):44-75, July 1994.

3. Bell, K. "Physician Profiling: 12 Critical Points." *Journal of Ambulatory Care Management* 19(1):81-5, Jan. 1996.

4. Bennett, G., and others. "Case Study in Physician Profiling." *Managed Care Quarterly* 2(4):60-70, Autumn 1994.

5. McKinney, L. "Paying for Quality." *Family Practice Management* 2(1):30-40, Jan. 1995.

6. Brand, D., and others. "Medical Practice Profiling: Concepts and Caveats." *Medical Care Research and Review* 52(2):223-51, June 1995.

7. McNeil, B., and others. "Current Issues in Profiling Quality of Care." *Inquiry* 29(3):298-307, Fall 1992.

8. Leatherman, S., and others. "Quality Screening and Management Using Claims Data in a Managed Care Setting." *Quality Review Bulletin* 17(11):349-59, Nov. 1991.

9. Risk Adjustment White Paper. Oak Brook, Ill.: University Hospital Consortium, 1991.

10. Iezzoni, L. "The Risks of Risk Adjustment." *JAMA* 278(19):1600-6, Nov. 19, 1997.

11. Hendryx, M., and others. "Using Comparative Clinical and Economic Outcome Information to Profile Physician Performance." *Health Services Management Research* 8(4):213-20, Nov. 8, 1995.

12. Tucker, A., and others. "Profiling Primary Care Physician Resource Use: Examining the Application of Case Mix Adjustment." *Journal of Ambulatory Care Management* 19(1):60-80, Jan. 1996.

13. Salem-Schatz, S., and others. "The Case for Case-Mix Adjustment in Practice Profiling-When Good Apples Look Bad." *JAMA* 272(11):871-4, Sept. 21, 1994.

14. Berlowitz, D., and others. "Ambulatory Care Case Mix Measures." *Journal of General Internal Medicine* 10(3):162-9, March 1995.

15. Roblin, D. "Patient Case Mix Measurement Using Outpatient Drug Dispense Data." *Managed Care Quarterly* 2(3):38-47, Summer 1994.

16. Greene, B., and others. "Ambulatory Care Groups and the Profiling of Primary Care Physician Resource Use: Examining the Application of Case Mix Adjustments." *Journal of Ambulatory Care Management* 19(1):86-9, Jan. 1996.

17. Starfield, B., and others. "Ambulatory Care Groups: A Categorization of Diagnoses for Research and Management." *Health Services Research* 26(1):53-74, April 1991.

18. Nugent, E. "Data Base Compares Productivity." *Medical Group Management Journal* 41(4):12-31, July-Aug. 1994.

19. Gray, J. *Evidence-Based Healthcare: How to Make Health Policy and Management Decisions.* London, England: Pearson Professional Limited, 1997.

20. Greco, P., and Eisenberg, J. "Changing Physician Practices-Commentary." *New England Journal of Medicine* 329(17):1271-4, Oct. 21, 1993.

21. Klein, L., and others. "Effects of Physician Tutorials on Prescribing Patterns of Graduate Physicians." *Journal of Medical Education* 56(6):504-11, June 1981.

22. Lomas, J., and others. "Opinion Leaders vs. Audit and Feedback to Implement Practice Guidelines: Delivery after Previous Cesarean Section." *JAMA* 265(17):2202-7, May 1, 1991.

23. Avorn, J., and Soumerai, S. "Improving Drug Therapy Decisions through Educational Outreach: A Randomized Controlled Trial of Academically Based "Detailing." *New England Journal of Medicine* 308(24):1457-63, June 16, 1983.

24. Covell, D., and others. "Information Needs in Office Practice: Are They Being Met?" *Annals of Internal Medicine* 103(4):596-9, Oct. 1985.

25. Kasper, J., and others. "Developing Shared Decision-Making Programs to Improve the Quality of Health Care." *Quality Review Bulletin* 18(6):183-90, June 1992.

26. Zander, K. "Nursing Case Management: Strategic Management of Cost and Quality Outcomes." *Journal of Nursing Administration* 18(5):23-30, May 1998.

27. Davis, D., and others. "Changing Physician Performance: A Systematic Review of the Effect of Continuing Medical Education Strategies." *JAMA* 274(9):700-5, Sept. 6, 1995.

28. Kassirer, J. "The Use and Abuse of Practice Profiles." *New England Journal of Medicine* 330(9):634-5, March 3, 1994.

29. Prager, L. "Profiling Gains Acceptance within Profession." *American Medical News* 40(18):4, May 12, 1997.

John B. Coombs, MD, is T.J. Phillips Professor of Family Medicine; Associate Vice President for Medical Affairs, Clinical Systems and Networks; and Associate Dean, Regional Affairs and Rural Health, Health Sciences Center, University of Washington School of Medicine, Seattle. Margaret H. Gilshannon, MHA, is Director, Clinical Systems Development, Health Sciences Center, University of Washington School of Medicine.

CHAPTER 6

The Legal Status of Provider Profiles
by Todd Sagin, MD, JD

*T*he evolution and nature of provider profiling is described at length throughout this monograph. The rapid growth in the generation of performance profiles and the multitude of uses to which such reports are put create a variety of opportunities for the accrual of liability. The classes of individuals who may feel injured by creation and dissemination of performance profiles includes patients, physicians, payers, and health care provider organizations. The perceived injury may come from unauthorized use of data to create a profile, the information portrayed by the profile, or the objectives to which the profile is applied. In recent years, collection of large databases of health care information has also led to increased concerns about privacy. "Data mining" and profiling can legitimately ignite fears about accuracy, privacy, security, and liability.

The health care community is rushing forward with profiling technology well ahead of any widely accepted ground rules-rules of behavior or of ethical conduct. This is the circumstance in which we frequently turn to our courts and judicial system to hammer out acceptable terms for the use of a technology. The legal system then works out the compromises necessary to accommodate the interests of multiple parties and to protect the rights of individuals.

This chapter will provide a general overview of some of the arenas in which profile use is likely to raise legal concerns. In particular, the concerns performance profiling raise around data confidentiality, credentialing, and medical malpractice will be explored. This chapter is designed to provide interested parties with only an overview of the issues involved. Rapidly evolving developments in health law will need assiduous monitoring by those responsible for protecting an organization and its individuals from the legal risks involved in performance analysis.

Malpractice Litigation

Physician concern that provider profiles will be utilized by plaintiff lawyers in malpractice suits has been voiced since the very first performance reports were made public. This same fear has been raised whenever some entity has promulgated medical standards, clinical practice guidelines, group benchmarks, or performance "report cards." The highly litigious atmosphere engulfing medical practice in recent decades renders these worries more than understandable. However, in recent years no avalanche of new malpractice suits based on such evidence has materialized.

Generally speaking, state law governs medical malpractice litigation. One way in which a state court might view performance profiles in litigation is as evidence of customary practice in the medical profession. In this regard, the performance profile is used in a similar fashion to a clinical practice guideline. The guideline serves as evidence of customary practice in the medical profession, and, in most jurisdictions, adherence to prevalent professional standards is an adequate defense to a medical negligence claim. Similarly, if a physician's performance profile reflects conformity with the common practice of peers, this may be sufficient evidence to undermine an assertion of malpractice. Of course the reverse circumstance can also occur. Here the plaintiff's attorney subpoenas profiling information that is then used to suggest that the physician had a pattern of negligent behavior-e.g., under-prescribing a medicine or under-utilization of screening tests. (These are frequently profiled behaviors and ones in which it is common for physicians to fail to meet national standards or standards promulgated by their provider groups or managed care organizations, MCOs).

When lawyers use a physician profile in this fashion, the profile (or guideline) acts more or less as an expert witness would, informing the court as to standard practice. The performance profile may be seen as more objective evidence than that offered by a witness and may prove more helpful or more damaging to the physician's defense. Lawyers may criticize the methodology and technique employed in creating the profile to cast doubt on the profile's accuracy. The issue of who generated the profile, what stature they hold in the professional world, what credibility their efforts have earned, and with what motivation they created the performance report, all may mitigate the impact a profile will have in litigation.

Another element affecting how a court might treat a profile in a given case reflects who is introducing the profile as evidence. Will the profile be more readily accepted as a piece of evidence in defense of practitioners or as a weapon in an attack on their competence? The evidence with regard to clinical guidelines may be instructive here. In general, such guidelines have been more effective as defense tools than in the armamentarium of the plaintiff attorney. An example is found in the 1990 Maine Medical Malpractice Demonstration Project, which clearly established the use of guidelines as a defense to the claim of malpractice and conversely restricted their use by plaintiffs.[1] The statute reads in part:

"§2975:Introduced by Plaintiff

In any claim for professional negligence against a physician...participating in the project...in which a violation of a standard of care is alleged, *only the physician*...may introduce into evidence as an affirmative defense, the existence of the practice parameters and risk management protocols developed and adopted [pursuant hereto]...for that medical specialty area."[2]

Minnesota, Kentucky, Florida, and Vermont have also taken this general approach.[3] This same tack could be found in the Clinton health system reform proposal, which, although dead, nevertheless contained many elements that reflect widespread thinking about health litigation issues.

Given the strong demand for "report cards" and profiles coming from the business community and from other purchasers of health care, it seems likely that political pressure will continue to mount to assure doctors that their compliance in this effort will not be turned to their detriment. However, it cannot be expected that, as physician profiles proliferate, they will be widely prohibited from use by plaintiff attorneys. Such a position flies in the face of basic fairness. Some states (e.g., Maryland) have resolved this concern with regard to clinical guidelines by not allowing them to be used as evidence by either side in a lawsuit.[4]

Can performance profiling reduce the number of lawsuits against physicians? If the data generated show a physician whose practice is in concert with his peers, suits might be discouraged. And if the ultimate goal of profiles to improve the quality of care is actually accomplished by such reports, justifiable lawsuits will diminish in response.

A recent use of data mining technology is the use of patient-specific data to create "risk appraisals" of specific patients. In this practice, an MCO, interested in targeting preventive measures at high-risk patients, profiles the patients of a specific practice and alerts the attending physicians to patients missing important preventive interventions. Some physicians have asked that the MCO, independent practice association (IPA), or other profiling entity not share data from such patient profiles with them, because it may create a legal obligation to act on the information. For example, there are attorneys who advise client organizations not to provide primary care physicians with patient-specific profiling data on mammography rates. The danger for the physician arises when he or she fails to act in a timely fashion upon notice that a specific patient has not had an indicated mammogram and the patient is subsequently found to have breast disease. This is an example where patient profiling puts the provider on notice of a need for intervention, and failure to take appropriate medical steps creates liability. Physicians must create systems to ensure that they document an adequate response to patient-specific profiling information that is shared with them. This situation is paralleled in the hospital setting when physician profiling puts the institution on notice of a potential quality problem with a medical staff member. This issue is discussed further later in this chapter.

Physicians are not the only individuals or entities that must be concerned about malpractice liability. Can lawsuits be brought against the parties creating a performance profile? The pressure to hold such individuals or organizations accountable will grow with the importance profiles play in the evolving health care marketplace. There are several potential theories under which such litigation might emerge. Negligence in creation of a profile or in its interpretation to the public might occur if incorrect or incomplete information is collected, the data are improperly analyzed, or if the data are assembled and presented in a misleading or an inaccurate manner. A negligence lawsuit might be filed if an injury to a patient results. If the harm of negligent profiling is to the business of another health care provider, legal action sounding in contract or intentional tort might result. Intentional torts can also raise the specter of punitive damages levied against the profiling entity that does so with intent to harm a competitor. Note, however, that if the profiling entity is a government body, a right of sovereign immunity may be applicable.

In the managed care context, the failure to track noncompliance or "outlier" performance with regard to clinical practice guidelines is a possible basis for establishing negligence. If profiling has demonstrated performance at variance with norms or standards, an injured plaintiff can argue that the harm incurred was a reasonably foreseeable consequence of the provider's behavior.[5] Not only managed care organizations, but also various provider organizations that take on utilization review and medical management functions may face similar consequences when they engage in the review of profiling data.

In the world of managed care organizations (MCOs), public frustration with cost control tactics has led plaintiffs to explore new ways to create liability for these companies and their employees. Techniques such as creation of clinical practice guidelines, performance profiles, and physician report cards place the health care insurer in the position of influencing the nature of a beneficiary's medical treatment. In contrast to the direct influence exerted by an MCO's utilization review department, the effects of performance profiles and related tools indirectly affect a physician's medical decisions. Beneficiaries are now promoting various legal theories that assert that payers have a legal responsibility to operate cost and quality control programs in a way that avoids medical harm. They are having increasing success holding insurers responsible for the malpractice of physicians whose treatment decisions are influenced by the actions of payers, even if that influence is indirect, as would be the case with a physician profile.

Providers and defendant organizations often claim that profiling information is privileged and cannot be introduced into evidence against them. However, much of the information requested in malpractice suits cannot be privileged because it is information collected in the "ordinary course of business." As profiling becomes more and more routine in large payer and provider organizations, it is an everyday part of managing the business. And the growing power of information technology makes the collection and analysis of such data increasingly easy to accomplish. This is a consequence of the increasing corporate nature of medicine. When discussing physician profiling, if talking about productivity, utilization rates, and clinical outcomes produced in the ordinary course of business, the data are not protected.

Confidentiality

The ability to assemble considerable amounts of information about patients and about providers will complement the shift toward more population-based approaches to preventive and chronic health care. One consequence is rising concern about who "owns" data and with whom data can be shared, both of which will be points of serious contention in the years ahead. Failure to craft careful policies with regard to the use of data essential to profiling can, at a minimum, lead to a public relations debacle. Most patients are not aware of the degree to which information from their insurance and medical records is collected and utilized in various profiling activities. It is likely many would object to having patient-specific information added to databases, either because of a perceived invasion of privacy or because they object to the ends to which the information is being used.

Most of the statutes and rules that govern the confidentiality of medical information were formulated years before sharing of such information to systematically improve quality management was contemplated. In today's models of health care, rigorous compliance with obsolete confidentiality laws cannot always be accomplished without sacrificing important management benefits created by clinical data repositories. Traditional patient authorizations for release of data are generally insufficient to authorize the kind of information sharing that is possible through data warehouses. These consent documents typically cover release of information for use in specific patient treatment or to acquire reimbursement but do not address additional quality and utilization control purposes. In addition, such patient authorizations are usually time limited, whereas the need of providers to access the data for profiling purposes is often ongoing. Some organizations have designed new "enterprise" authorizations that define a much broader set of uses for the patient's data. Users of medical data repositories should be required to sign appropriate user agreements that commit them to confidentiality parameters and that have a mechanism to terminate their privileges if they are abused.

Performance data are often produced from claims information in payer databases. When provider groups seek these data from payers in order to profile physician behavior, what, if any, consent must be obtained directly from the patient? At present, there is no clear answer to this question, and actual practice by payers and their affiliated clinical groups varies tremendously. Many insurers have begun to consider and draft restrictive policies governing the use of their claims data. This may be frustrating for providers and MCO medical directors who seek information to improve quality of care, but it is probably prudent action from a risk management perspective. It should also be viewed as an ethically correct course of action until adequate guidelines for the use of health care data are vetted and accepted.

Numerous states require some type of accountability from health plans for quality. In addition some states require payers to achieve some type of accreditation for their utilization activities. Organizations such as the National Committee for Quality Assurance (NCQA), the Utilization Review and Accreditation Commission (URAC), and the Joint Commission for the Accreditation of Healthcare Organizations (JCAHO) carry out accreditation activities and generally require health plans to aggregate data that can demonstrate "quality." Health plans, in turn, require physicians to provide, or allow to be used, data about their practices and practice patterns. There is wide diversity in the way in which these health plans collect and acquire data. A health plan will typically argue that the patient "belongs" to them and that they have a legitimate claim on information concerning the patient. The concept that his or her treating provider or health plan owns an individual's medical information is rooted in property law. Most subscribers sign a release of information when they enroll with a health plan, consenting to disclosure of information necessary for the administration of the health insurance benefit. In a society increasingly aware of the sensitivity of information, these clauses may be challenged in the future as unlawful. Most states have adopted statutes that limit the type of information that can be shared (with limitations on HIV, mental health, or treatment of substance abuse the most likely restrictions). Increasingly, disclosure agreements are expected to be time-sensitive and time-specific in their delineation of the information that can be shared.

Sometimes the burden lies with the doctor to acquire patients' consent to have information from their records shared with an MCO creating profiles. Occasionally, a health plan will assert that it has obtained such patient consent and will even indemnify the physician if he or she discloses in reliance on this claim and it is subsequently determined that the consent is invalid.

In some areas, managed care organizations delegate quality of care monitoring to an IPA, an integrated delivery system (IDS), or another provider organization. These organizations then require the MCO's data in order to carry out quality initiatives through provider profiling. The information they need is often patient-specific claims information and thus carries a particular sensitivity. Agreements should exist between the payer and the provider organizations that specify how such information can be utilized and what confidentiality protections must be in place.

The information ownership claims of health providers and payers will likely be attenuated over the next several years as the federal government develops and institutes regulations to implement the privacy and security mandates of the Health Insurance Portability and Accountability Act of 1996 (P.L.104-191, also referred to as HIPAA). This law will clarify individuals' rights over medical information and strip health plans and providers of some of the rights they have asserted to control medical data sets. HIPAA may create a much-needed national game plan for health information security and privacy. This should result in an improvement over the current situation, in which privacy rights are left to a plethora of state and federal laws and to a general obligation on the part of providers to protect patient "confidentiality." Under HIPAA, if Congress fails to enact federal health information privacy legislation by August 21, 1999, the Secretary of Health and Human Service is required to promulgate final regulations containing privacy standards applicable to financial and administrative transactions subject to HIPAA's standards by February 21, 2000. These final regulations will supersede all contrary provisions of state law, except those imposing more stringent requirements or standards.

The potential of profiling and other sensitive health information to course through the Internet has likewise gotten the attention of the federal government. The Internet currently is largely unregulated and ungoverned. High levels of security are being required to avoid disastrous breaches of patient or provider confidentiality. Although most of the attention currently is focused on protecting patient information that is shared across the Internet, similar sensitivity is required for provider profiles being distributed across this increasingly valuable communications medium.

Medical personnel dealing with information management should not overlook the government's recent aggressive posture toward enforcement of federal health care laws. Confidentiality concerns may turn out to be one of the most serious areas of compliance exposure for physicians and health care executives. Indeed, criminal penalties are now being contemplated to enforce law dealing with confidentiality issues. The American Health Information Management Association (AHIMA), a national organization of health information management professionals, is generally a good source of information on developments in this area.

A number of state governments have set up agencies for the purpose of collecting health care data and creating physician and payer profiles. Where this is the case, state statutes and regulations protect the process of data accumulation and may spell out responsibilities for preservation of data confidentiality. States use the collated information in a variety of ways, including generation of "report cards" and profiles. However, they generally do not collect patient-specific data and therefore avoid dealing with the most sensitive confidentiality concerns.

Credentialing

Liability may exist for organizations, physicians, or administrative personnel who profile provider performance for purposes of hospital or managed care network credentialing. Credentialing, long a hospital-based responsibility, has become a hallmark activity of managed care organizations, and it is one of their primary quality assurance activities. Extensive information is gathered on the provider being credentialed, and generally the provider must consent to its use for this purpose if he or she wishes to contract with the payer. Employers and the public are increasingly aware of this review procedure and its role in network provider selection/participation. Profiles of physicians, based on information ostensibly gathered for credentialing purposes, now find their way into health plan directories, marketing materials, and accreditation surveys.

When a physician agrees to a credentialing procedure, whether by a hospital or a health plan, he or she generally waives the right to privacy of the information gathered. When a physician signs an application or payer contract, more often than not he or she has agreed to allow investigation of:

■ Work history.

■ Physical and mental health as it pertains to the ability to deliver health care.

■ Records at other institutions, including quality reports and any performance profiles that may have been created.

Such applications or contracts usually contain a specific release for accumulation of these data, and some will require the doctor to waive a right to sue for
defamation or invasion of privacy. (This waiver is valid only as long as the credentialing investigation is carried out properly and without malice.)

One tactic by which provider groups may be able to shield their profiling data
is to claim that it is protected if it has been used in a peer review process. In
many cases, peer protection laws (which sprung up in the mid-1970s during
one of the recurring national malpractice crises) shield from legal liability and
damage awards physicians engaged in review of their colleagues' attributes and
work. The rationale for these laws is that such protection is necessary in order
to ensure promotion of high-quality medical care. These laws tend to create
protections of two sorts. The first are confidentiality shields, protecting the
information submitted to relevant committees from being introduced as evidence in medical malpractice litigation. The second are immunity provisions,
which shield physicians acting in good faith on such committees from lawsuits
brought by doctors who are sanctioned via the peer review process.

These "peer review" laws were initially created for hospital credentialing activities, and most states did not include payers within the ambit of these protections.
Similarly, the laws rarely address the activities of nonhospital provider organizations, such IPAs, physician-hospital organizations (PHOs), or IDS. In some
case law, courts have ordered the disclosure by an HMO of information that
would otherwise be considered protected if created by a "provider."[6] However,
these organizations protect themselves through the inclusion of waiver and
immunity provisions in their application forms, thereby creating contractually
protections that may not be available under state peer protection acts.

The federal Health Care Quality Improvement Act of 1986 (HCQIA) also creates a privilege for peer review processes. Although this statute has generally
been used to create a safe harbor for credentialing, it may also protect some
profiling activities-especially when used as part of a recredentialing or a quality assurance process. In accordance with HCQIA, profiling data should be protected when they are disclosed in a peer review meeting and to people involved
in the peer review program. Such a committee may meet regularly to review
and discuss profiling data. The peer review committee might look at quality
assurance information that comes from the profiles-e.g., mammogram rates,
newly diagnosed cancer rates, or mortality rates for each physician in a
provider group. All of that information should be protected from plaintiff attorneys under peer review law. HCQIA is a seminal piece of federal legislation

enacted to increase access across the country to information about poor physician performers. Organizations gathering data on doctors and wishing protection from antitrust and defamation suits when they reject such physicians for affiliation must report their decisions to the National Practitioner Data Bank. This action becomes another way in which outside parties may become aware of the likely existence of negative physician profiling data. If an organization takes actions toward a physician but does not report them to the National Practitioner Data Bank, a privilege of confidentiality may be lost. The federal law clearly specifies the way to handle such reporting. If there is deviation, privilege over any information used in the peer review process, including profiling data, is lost.

Profiling may be a critical issue where claims of negligent credentialing are alleged. In *Cronic v. Doud*,[5] the fact that a hospital supposedly had a utilization review program in place was critical to the claim of liability. The surgeon had a pattern of inappropriate surgeries based on misdiagnosis of thoracic outlet syndrome. All six such patients seen by the doctor had bad outcomes. The critical issue allowing the plaintiffs to move forward with their case was that the hospital had notice that the surgeon had a problem. The court noted that the hospital was put on notice by its monitoring of the numbers and the types of surgeries and that it should have responded to the data with an investigation of the physician involved in this case. In this case, the court asserted that performance profiling created enough evidence of a potential problem that the hospital was negligent in not further investigating the appropriateness of this physician's surgical privileges.

Economic Credentialing

The activity of provider performance analysis has created from its start significant consternation among physicians, who fear abuse of the information gathered. Historically, doctors have carried out their work with little scrutiny, and the use of early profiling to support "economic credentialing" efforts heightened their suspicion that this was a tool destined for "misuse." This practice, wherein a payer or a provider organization attempts to remove or exclude a physician from its delivery network when he or she fails to meet economic expectations, may be justified on the basis of performance reports created from the data collection efforts of the MCO.

Information sought from providers typically includes data for quality assurance and utilization management activities. However, in an era in which provider groups are increasingly put at significant financial risk, various players have a clear interest in financial information as well. Donald Rickabaugh, MD, a southern California physician, filed a lawsuit against the Greater Newport Physicians Group in Newport Beach, California, and PacifiCare Health

Systems, Inc., of Santa Ana, California. The suit was brought in concert with an advocacy group called Consumers for Quality Care in Santa Monica, California. The suit claims that Rickabaugh was terminated because of poor performance on the HMO's pharmacy profiles, which compared physicians' prescription drug costs. This is an example of a claim that asserts profiling information has been used to demonstrate a physician does not contribute adequately to the bottom line of an MCO or a provider group. The profile becomes justification for eliminating the physician from participation in an HMO's provider network, an IPA, or a group practice.

The attorneys working on behalf of the defendants say Rickabaugh was dismissed from the group after audits showed his medical office was operated in a grossly substandard manner and after several patient complaints had been received. These attorneys claim that the cost profiles were not determinative of this doctor's dismissal from the IPA. However, after being given written and oral notice of the problems, a decision was made that Rickabaugh could not cure the concerns enumerated.[7]

The case and statutory law regarding economic credentialing is voluminous, and an extensive literature exists analyzing this practice. For purposes of this review, suffice it to note that, when creating provider performance profiles, it is wise to clearly articulate, through written policies, the uses to which the information can be put. This puts all parties on notice regarding the intentions of those with control over the profiling reports. To the degree that it is an accurate reflection of the profiler's intent, a goal of improving the quality and the efficiency of care should always be emphasized as foremost in importance.

Trade Libel

Trade libel is publication to third parties of a false statement that disparages an individual's products or services and results in pecuniary loss to that individual. The dissemination of provider or group-specific profiling information has the potential to cause significant economic harm to the profiled parties. Whether the injured provider is a solo practitioner, a group practice, or a large health system, it may believe that it is suffering from an unfair and malicious portrait of its work. A plaintiff asserting a claim of trade libel needs to prove five elements to make a case.

- Publication to a third party.

- A false statement of fact.

- The third party's understanding that the statement is derogatory.

■ Malice.

■ Damages.

The danger of trade libel arises in today's highly competitive health care marketplaces where assertions of quality are increasingly the currency of public marketing campaigns. Those producing provider profiles that may be used in this manner must be scrupulous as to the methodological accuracy of their profiling reports and assure themselves that they can legitimately assert objectivity in their work. To prevail with a trade libel claim, a plaintiff must prove that the profiles in question constitute false assertions of fact. Where profiling is done with the intent of improving quality of care, and not as a duplicitous exercise in bashing a marketplace opponent, fear of a trade libel action need not be a significant concern.

Entities that are targets of direct government regulation, such as HMOs and PPOs, are sometimes subject to specific advertising proscriptions that may limit the ways in which they can use profiling information. IDSs, IPAs, and other health care organizations that are less regulated will still find that state and federal laws address unfair trade practices. The Federal Trade Commission acts to enforce these laws at the federal level and to protect organizations against unfair methods of competition. The Lanham Act[8] provides for a private right of action as well as injunctive remedies to parties that believe they have been victims of deceptive advertising. This act was invoked by two large insurers in the Philadelphia marketplace, who went to court over competing claims as to which payer delivers better value in health care delivery and insurance.[9]

In *Healthnet v. Weiss Research Inc.*, a 1994 California case,[10] an HMO brought suit against a financial rating organization when it was dissatisfied with the ranking it received in the company's published report on HMO financial security. The HMO sought an injunction against the publication of the rating company's "report card" as well as unspecified financial damages. If the defendant had been ranking the physician performance of various HMOs, a similar suit might have been asserted.

Those who wish to use physician profiles as a tool in advertising and to gain marketplace advantage should seek out competent legal counsel to ensure they are engaging in a legally permissible business tactic.

Fraud and Abuse Investigations

Federal and state governments have committed enormous resources to combat fraud in the health care field. One increasing use of physician profiling is to track patterns that indicate submission of fraudulent Medicare or other insurance claims. By looking at patterns of provider behavior, investigators can target candidates for further scrutiny. Providers should be aware that, when they release data for use by others to profile, it might be used to ensure that they are in compliance with federal and state laws. We will likely see profiles that suggest improper or illegal behavior used as evidence in government criminal fraud cases. One example of a statute supporting such use of profiles is the previously mentioned Health Insurance Portability and Accountability Act of 1996 (HIPAA), which amends the Civil Money Penalties portion of the Fraud and Abuse Act to hold physicians liable for a "pattern of medically unnecessary billings.[11]

Suggestions to Reduce the Risk of Liability

■ Profiles should be developed in accordance with commonly accepted methodological and evaluative procedures wherever possible. An explanation should be available on how they were developed and what proper conclusions can be drawn from them. In addition, information should be available on limitations regarding conclusions that can be drawn from the profile. Profiles should incorporate some level of severity or risk adjustment whenever possible, and the rigor of this adjustment should be explicated in the dissemination of the profile data.

■ Avoid sharing profile information that contains any patient-specific information. Accepted ethical parameters and increasingly strict statutory and regulatory proscriptions should provide ample motivation to keep patient data anonymous. Care must be taken to ensure that the database- and computer-savvy individual cannot uncover patient identifiers without proper authorization.

■ The primary use of physician profiles should be to enhance quality of care. The use of such reports for the sole purpose of cost control or the application of financial incentives to providers will incur higher risk of lawsuit.

■ If profiling information is meant to be used solely for credentialing or peer review activity, it should be kept strictly confidential and not be disclosed to parties not privy to the protections of the peer review process. An organization can lose its peer review protections if information is given to people who are not part of the peer review process. Once the information is given to someone whose access to it is not privileged, the information itself will no longer be considered privileged. Where broader dissemination does occur, it should be done only when provider identifiers have been removed. If guests are present at peer review meetings, information that is shared must be blinded. Additionally, guests should be asked to sign confidentiality statements. Indeed, all committee members should sign such statements when joining the group.

■ As a general observation, judges do not like to keep information out of the courtroom, and they exhibit a bias against privilege claims. One should deal with profiling information with a realization that it very well may end up in a courtroom.

■ Avoid using physician profiles for advertising purposes. Where such profiling is intended for use in competitive jockeying, seek review of the tactic from legal counsel familiar with the law governing fair trade practices.

The sophistication with which physician profiling is being performed is growing by leaps and bounds. There is every reason to expect that this will become a highly pervasive health care activity with potential to greatly affect the practice of health care in America. It is precisely because of its power as a tool for modifying provider behavior that we will inevitably see a bevy of legal cases emerge around the practice. This should be a reason to proceed with care and caution in the creation and use of physician profiles. However, it is unlikely that litigation or its threat will seriously deter this important trend. The prudent physician and health care executive, aware of the potential danger spots, should be able to proceed with physician profiling confident that he or she can safely employ it to enhance the quality of the medical care delivered.

References

1. "Professional Liability: Maine's Experiment with Practice Guidelines Produces Little Evidence," *Health Law Rep.* (BNA) 753,754 (June 9, 1994).

2. Maine Revised Statues Annotated, secs.2971-78(1990).

3. Minnesota Statute ß62J.34(3)(a)(1994); Kentucky Revised Statute Ann.342.035; Vermont Acts 160, ß 46, Florida Statute Ann. Sec.408.02.

4. Maryland Code Ann. [Health-Gen.] Sec.19-1606 (1995).

5. *Cronic v. Doud.* 168 Ill. App.3d 665, 523 NE 2d 176 (1988).

6. *McClellan v. Hempsey* 442 Pa. Super 504,660 A.2d 97 (1995).

7. Donald Rickabaugh, MD, a southern California physician, filed a lawsuit against the Greater Newport Physicians Group in Newport Beach, California, and PacifiCare Health Systems, Inc., of Santa Ana, California.

8. 15 USC § 1051 *et seq.*

9. *US Healthcare Inc. v. Blue Cross*, 898 F 2d 914, 916 (3d Cir. 1990).

10. *Healthnet v. Weiss Research Inc.*

11. 42 U.S.C. 1320a-7a(a)(1)(E).

Todd Sagin, MD, JD, is Senior Medical Director, Penn Care, Doylestown, Pennsylvania.

CHAPTER 7

The Informatics of
Physician Profiling

by David M. Klubert, MD, and Colt G. Courtright, MPA

*T*he authors' purpose in this chapter is to share the knowledge we have gained in developing central analysis capacities and incorporating new technology (and, in some cases, not-yet-developed technology) as part of a medical organization's efforts to meet the information demands of the 21st Century. Our intent is to add to readers' understanding of how information may be captured and integrated to enhance an organization's analytical and predictive capabilities.

We begin with some of the difficulties inherent in using analytical groupings to examine data collected for specific (and often incompatible) purposes and audiences. The influences that funding, statistical phenomena, and past information needs have had on the usefulness of existing databases and analyses are presented in this section.

Then we review the need for data integration across care environments. The importance of wholistic examinations of data for the ability to accurately assess medical practices and outcomes is discussed.

Efforts to incorporate control mechanisms in existing grouping methodologies through the use of case-mix, severity, environment, disease, and other adjustments are then presented. Here, the authors discuss the differences among adjustment mechanisms developed since 1985.

Finally, we make predictions about the future evolution of severity adjustment modeling. Arguments are made for changing the existing interpretation of disease from diagnosis or diagnostic groupings to symptoms, physiological variables, and quantified outcomes, as well as for incorporating treatment algorithms to operationalize research and policy-level findings.

Shortcomings to Historical Uses of Information

Human beings enjoy bringing order to chaos. The need to track spending led to the creation of accounting departments; the desire to expand market share led to demographic profiling; the need to retain existing customers led to the use of satisfaction surveys and customer profiling analyses; and the identification of new biological phenomena led to the creation of new testing instruments. The underlying premise here is that *cause* led to *effect*; that *action* led to reaction; and that, in many instances, these reactions perpetuate themselves.

The result of this evolutionary development, except for cases in which strategic planning has taken place, is that information commonly is collected and used for past purposes. The ability to perform current and future analysis is affected by past needs, as exhibited through current delineations of data. Data collection therefore frequently is characterized by what have become known as Finagle's Laws: "The data you want are not the data you have; the data you have are not the data you need; the data you need are not the data you can afford; and the data you can afford are not the data you want."[1]

Unfortunately, these "laws" are largely reflective of reality. Data collection efforts cost money, so they are conducted for specific purposes. Expansion of analyses or interpretation beyond these purposes is difficult, if not impossible, and organizations suffer from information stratification. Current grouping methods and their shortcomings are described below.

Inheritors of Evolutionary Data Systems

Data commonly are grouped around a specific purpose. Data may be grouped for measurement against past performance, against the performance of similar efforts, or against some specific goal. Data collection may be designed around either global or local applicability needs. Data collection efforts may be designed to corroborate existing beliefs (confirmatory analysis) or to identify new, unknown, or unpredicted phenomena (exploratory analysis).

Regardless of how or why data are collected, information inherently is grouped around some purpose. Research methodology and economics both show that this is appropriate—data collection without a specific hypothesis/purpose is misguided and wasteful of fixed resources. Contemporary methodology tells us that we should clearly identify who or what is to be studied (the unit of analysis), how the changes in the unit of analysis are to be measured (measures of analysis), and the means by which the investigation effort is to be assessed (rejection or acceptance of null hypotheses).

A dominant underlying reason for the traditional approach is that information costs money. The traditional approach is given further impetus by the statistical phenomenon that the smaller the variations within each group (the more homogeneous the group), the easier it is to identify differences between groups with fewer observations. Fewer observations mean fewer collection efforts and, therefore, reduced research costs.

This means that, if the desired information can be made sufficiently specific to enable populations to be chosen more diligently (with a more homogeneous membership), the ability to distinguish (test for significant differences) between groups using smaller populations will be increased. Therefore, there are financial incentives to conduct analyses for only premeditated purposes, as well as to increase the specificity of each purpose.

Captured Audience Syndrome

Grouping of data in health care organizations, as in most other organizations, frequently revolves around the consumer audience for each specific area of the business. Information grouped for financial administrators may make little physiologic sense. Conversely, the information used by doctors is largely clinically derived and may not pertain to any concept of financial performance. As a result, those who are responsible for patient well-being have little knowledge of efficient allocations of effort, and those who are administering resources are largely unable to communicate the relative physiologic trade-offs of alternative expenditures. Because groupings are seldom standardized, a direct assessment of relative contributions to patient care and disease costs is not possible. Further, the relative impact that decisions at various points of the care spectrum have on outcomes and costs are never known at the patient, demographic group, or disease levels—at least not without specialized investigations.

Administrators and researchers are all too aware of the implications of this scenario—each agency sees a part of the spectrum of care but is unaware of the level, quality, or constitution of other efforts. The authors believe that the lack of a crosswalk or a uniform measure by which communication can travel is a dangerous phenomenon as we move toward HMO networks in this country.

Comparison Categories: Beginning the Systemization Trend

Efforts to develop consistent groupings across organizations have begun. An obvious example is the diagnosis-related group (DRG) payment system implemented in the early 1980s. This system allows hospitals to make local or national comparisons of their DRG mixes. Similarly, relative value units (RVUs) allow comparisons across institution boundaries and provide some indication of the need to allocate additional resources to physiologic conditions. HEDIS indicators enable qualitative comparisons across managed care organizations using uniform groupings. Many HMOs use logical groupings of provider types (internal medicine, family practice, obstetrics, etc.) that, with local agreements, can be shared with others to gather information about performance. For obvious reasons, tracking by contractual arrangements also takes place.

A number of shortcomings to existing grouping mechanisms, noted by many authors elsewhere, remain. We will briefly mention only two of the deficits.

■ First, the information used in the groupings is predominantly payment-based. Because payment systems are largely based on provided services, not on the symptoms for which the services are provided, much medically relevant information is lost. Interactive and additive effects of multiple illnesses/diseases frequently cannot be assessed. Moreover, many of the procedures performed on a patient may not even relate to the diagnosis itself. (For instance, preventive and diagnostic services such as immunizations, laboratory tests, etc., are commonly separate from the primary reason a patient seeks medical attention.) Hence, groupings around this information are highly inaccurate.

■ Second, information presently collected to understand cost, quality (HEDIS), and effort (RVUs) does not account for differences among physicians, among local and regional provider groups, or in the severity of the illnesses of patients. The fact that costs are higher than elsewhere or are rising rapidly over previous numbers may reflect poor decision making on the part of physicians or more severely ill patients. Patterns observed in existing groupings do not enable management organizations to understand observed data patterns or to develop policies and guidelines to modify clinical behavior.

Data Integration along the Health Care Continuum

At the beginning of this section, the authors would like to propose four concepts:

■ Economies of scale exist in data collection efforts.

■ Economies of scale exist in data management.

■ Economies of scale exist in report generation.

■ Significant incidental savings exist in integrating data across health care environments.

There are economies of scale in data collection efforts. Most health care facilities work with a number of clinicians, oversight bodies, physician management groups, and external specialist providers. If data are to be shared between these groups to individually track clientele, all providers along any given patient's care continuum must exchange information. Each organization must have the technical support necessary to integrate information received from all other partners. A more cost-efficient alternative, assuming that organizations on average have fewer operating systems than they have health care partners, is to have a central data integration organization. In this way, system conversion and integration programs would have to be created only once. Further, when any facility changes operating systems or software, changes to integration have to be made only once—not once for each information sharer.

There also are economies of scale in data management. Knowledge about individual data elements would not need to be retained in multiple sites, but merely in a central data management structure. In this way, the arduous effort to ensure that "apples" are compared to other "apples" would not need to be duplicated.

Finally, there are economies of scale in report generation. The ability to automate reports through custom programming software (i.e., SAS[2]) implies that uniform information may be provided over time. This uniform information has lower maintenance costs over time, while the initial set-up costs may be distributed across large production volumes. If customized formats can be forsaken for agreement about report content, agencies that do not have inherent analytical capabilities can operate far less blindly. Further, organizations with analytical components can focus their attention on analysis rather than on data integration and redundant report generation.

Note, however, that the advent of virtual data warehousing and browser technology is providing the possibility for new forms of organizational development. Economies of scale need not result in either the isolation or the joint positioning of data collection, management, and reporting (although there may be qualitative considerations that dictate a close relationship). Today, technology allows large integrated data structures within the following arrangements:

■ Local data storage and centralized reporting.

■ Centralized data storage and local reporting (querying).

■ Local data storage and local reporting.

■ Centralized data storage and centralized reporting.

Significant incidental savings also exist in integrating data across health care environments. Not the least of these benefits is the shift from individual entities pursuing organizational efficiency to entities pursuing social (or at least group) economic efficiency. With integration of data, contracts can be built around the

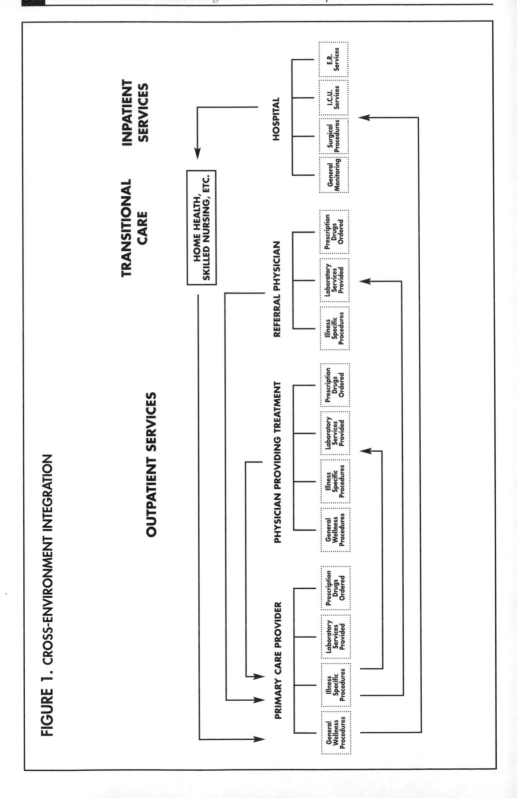

FIGURE 1. CROSS-ENVIRONMENT INTEGRATION

concept of reducing total care costs, thereby increasing the profit margins of individual entities.

Cross-Environment Data Integration

Tracking a patient along the continuum of medical care requires cross-purpose, cross-environment, cross-institution, and integration of data over time. Systemized downloads of raw data must take place to satisfy multiple purposes and consumers, each of which wants some specific evaluative or analytical interpretability. All pertinent outpatient, inpatient, pharmaceutical, and ancillary service information needs to be available for wholistic evaluation of care. A few of the benefits to such a system are illustrated by the feedback loops presented in figure 1, page 106.

Under most HMO schemes, primary care providers (or primary care clinics) are responsible for the health care services used by patient subpopulations. Our analyses have indicated, however, that any given primary care provider's (PCP's) subpopulation often is seen by physicians other than the PCP. Once the patient is referred to another site, the PCP frequently has little or no knowledge about further care decisions. In addition, the clinician is seldom aware of changes in prescribed medications based on a pharmacist's decisions or a patient's economic choices. One result of information integration across care environments is that providers all along the care spectrum can know on average (if not in each specific case) the implications of previous and later medical treatment decisions.

Filling the Information Gaps

For integrated information to be useful for allocating resources to medical problems, it must be complete. The condition of any given patient can be made dramatically better or significantly worse with a single medical procedure or service. The condition of patients and/or the outcome of medical services also may be influenced by decisions not captured. For instance, medical treatment foregone or utilized through advice nurses and phone consultations with physicians may significantly affect future treatment decisions, cost of care, and patient outcome. If we are to track patients individually or in groups, all information must be made available, systematically exported, and integrated within electronic media.

Implicit in the arguments for tracking all information is the authors' belief that the level of detail available for review needs to be increased. Lab tests and biopsy results, radiation dosage/frequency, and many other factors are not universally tracked in an electronic environment. Other physiologic factors, including specific measurements, rates of growth/development, etc., also are not captured in many instances. Time components, by which procedural order may be evaluated, are not routinely tracked, particularly in the outpatient world. To analyze data with accuracy will require creation of new units of observation and collection instruments and their linkage to sophisticated electronic tracking mechanisms.

To efficiently and effectively allocate resources, uniform measures of output and outcomes need to be developed. The RAND Corporation, through its Health Insurance Experiment and its Medical Outcomes Study, has provided a number of valid indicators of qualitative outcomes. Measures of social and emotional well-being have been created and integrated into such collection instruments as SF-36 and HSQ-12. Duke University has developed measures of patient satisfaction and physician evaluation to assess the likelihood of medical resource usage.[3] Still others, including the Health Outcomes Institute, have created condition-specific outcomes indicators. And last, but not least, there are those who are trying to create a uniformly acceptable definition of "outcomes" to enable further research to produce more applicable measures.[4]

An additional hurdle many researchers are trying to leap is the concept of risk adjustment or patient illness severity. Once information is integrated and can be analyzed in a holistic manner against acceptable outcomes, evaluators still will face the undeniable problem of disease or case severity. Even where patients have the same diagnosis applied to them by the same physician (and receive the same care), there likely will be different costs and medical outcomes associated with each patient. The same disease can strike different people in different ways, can affect individual anatomic systems differently, and can have varying levels of symptom intensity.

Incorporating Severity Controls and Methods of Evaluation

The assumption underlying all the differences in approaches to severity adjustment is that it is fundamentally important to know if patients are more severely ill in particular geographic regions, in demographic groups, or under particular treatment approaches. This is true from the perspective of policy formation and resource allocation; and physician management and profiling. The availability of information, combined with different audience needs, has led to the development of a number of severity-adjustment mechanisms. Each of these mechanisms perform adequately for a specific purpose, but not as well for more widely focused analyses.

Alternative Models of Severity Adjustment

Most of the severity-adjustment tools can be modeled on five scales:

■ Resource-based (administrative) vs. physiologically-based (clinical) severity adjustment.

■ Prediction of costs/resource use versus medical/physiological outcomes.

■ Applicability to retrospective versus prospective analysis.

■ The degree to which technology versus human resources must be used to gather data.

■ Single-environment vs. cross-environment orientation.

Resource-Based versus Physiology-Based Severity Adjustment

Severity-adjustment models have evolved to provide one of two different types of information—clinical or financial. Intensive care unit models are good examples of using clinical indicators to estimate physiologic outcomes. The Acute Physiology and Chronic Health Evaluation (APACHE II) system uses 12 physiologic variables, weighted using expert opinions, to derive a score and/or probability of mortality.[5-7] Similarly, the Simplified Acute Physiology Score (SAPS)[8] and Mortality Probability Models (MPM) systems use indicators such as the Glasgow Coma Scale and the existence of metastatic cancer to derive severity scores and probabilities of survival.[9-12] Others, including the Organ-System Failure (OSF) model, take into account physiologic changes over time.[13]

Moving across the spectrum toward models that attempt to provide information on resource intensity (LOS, inpatient costs, etc.) are models that use physiologic/diagnostic variables to estimate or predict cost streams for patient subpopulations (or, in the extreme, predict costs for a specific patient). The development of diagnosis-related groups (DRGs) for hospital reimbursement is an obvious example. Despite having a foundation in medical science, their use for reimbursement implies that it is driven by actuarial and financial concerns. As a result, DRGs' ability to define homogeneous groups of patients is hampered by the level of intra- and extra-class variation in resource usage. Others in this class include the Computerized Severity Index (CSI)[14,15] and New Jersey DRGs.

Further along the resource spectrum are models that concentrate on grouping total costs (i.e., pharmaceutical, optometry, laboratory/pathology, etc.) to identify resource usage patterns in the course of physician profiling and disease management associated with specific clinical decisions. These models generally examine data from productivity and financial viewpoints. Examples of these models include Diagnostic Episode Cluster (DEC)[16-19] and Episode Treatment Group (ETG)[20] methodologies. Finally, there are models that use statistical techniques or patient-reported (survey) information to develop categories of cost and resource use. These models tend to produce probable cost relationships to decisions and the influence of risk factors by defining homogeneous treatment/cost groups, rather than using physiological indications of severity or projected mortality.

Prediction of Costs/Resource Use versus Medical/Physiological Outcomes

The accuracy of alternative grouping models is partially explained by the previously discussed mechanisms. Models that are at the physiologic end of the severity-adjustment mechanism tend to have the highest degree of predictive accuracy for physiologic conditions (e.g., mortality). For instance, increase in mortality predictiveness over chance (C = 0.5) is much greater in the ICU models than in the inpatient models. Multiple observers have found ICU models to have C statistics that fall between .80 and .90.[21] This is compared to C statistics in the .60s and .70s for inpatient models.[22] This trend also is seen between the inpatient and outpatient models. Outpatient models (not predicting mortality) have been found to be characterized by C statistics in the high .50s and low .60s.[3]

On the other hand, the physiology-based models seem to be weaker in terms of explaining the variance in resource use than models directly based in resource intensity. DRGs have been found to account for 5 to 52 percent of hospital costs (generally around 20 percent), while ICU models account for substantially less.[23]

The physiology-based models also tend to be more consistent across models and research studies than resource intensity-based models. For example, Le Gall *et al.* identified actual-expected probability ratios of .73 to 1.31 across ICU units when using the SAPS II system.[8] In an evaluation of the APACHE II system, Knaus *et al.* found actual-expected probability ratios to vary across ICU units in the range of .67 to 1.25 for mortality and of .88 to 1.21 for length of stay.[21] Conversely, Iezzoni *et al.* found that DRGs accounted for 23-52 percent of the variation in hospital costs,[24] while Tierney *et al.* found that DRGs accounted for 16-25 percent of cost variance.[25]

Studies also have demonstrated that combining resource-based groupings with physiology-based groupings improves the ability to account for resource variation. Iezzoni *et al.* showed that the explained proportion of LOS variance across Medicare patients can be improved from 1-12 percent using MedisGroups to 9-41 percent using MedisGroups within DRGs.[26] Similarly, Horn *et al.* found that using the CSI within ADRGs improved the reduction in within-group variance to 28 percent, in comparison to 11 percent when using the CSI (at the time of admittance) alone.[14]

Applicability to Retrospective versus Prospective Analysis

Grouping models developed thus far range from those that must be applied prospectively to those that may be applied to past data collection and recording efforts. Prospective models generally require integration of new data collection instruments. These models also require staff training in identification of interrelationships across medical specialty lines (such as the adverse reaction to a drug prescribed by another/previous physician, in terms of its probable influence on a particular organ). These models also may require subjective determination of different levels of severity. Examples of prospective models include SF-36, HSQ-12 and DUKE/DUSOI, among others.

Models that enable retrospective analysis generally are not based on physician ratings, but rather on a process of associating key pieces of routinely collected information (procedure and diagnosis codes, length of episodes of care, associated or derivative comorbidities, etc.). For instance, the CSI uses discharge abstract information; DRGs use routinely collected procedure and surgical codes; and simple age/sex adjustments may be incorporated from nearly any recorded information. Today, the grouping process for models that apply preset criteria to existing/past data are automated.

The Degree to Which Technology versus Human Resources Must Be Used

This fourth spectrum on which alternative adjustment models may be placed reflects the trade-off in resources necessary to implement such systems. Early models of many systems were labor intensive, but most have graduated to the automated environment. The CSI, DRG, ACG, DEC, ETG, and Staging methodologies now are automated to greater or lesser extents. Others, such as the DUKE, SF-36, HSQ-12, and other survey-based methodologies continue to rely more heavily on the use of human resources. Those that rank highly on the resource end of the spectrum also require more patient participation, adding additional labor components to the collection process.

Single-Environment vs. Cross-Environment Orientation

Nearly all of the severity/treatment adjustment models have, until recently, been developed for, and applied to, particular markets and care environments. Most models were developed for inpatient hospital use, some for general tracking, and others for tracking specific cost centers (ICUs, EDs, etc.). Because the dominant basis for categorizing patients was (and is) the DRG payment system, very few models have developed to systematically define patient groups in the outpatient world. Physician profiling in the outpatient world traditionally has been limited to either raw data comparisons or case-mix adjusted comparisons, in which case mix is defined as age-sex adjustment.

Developments that have improved outpatient profiling include the Medical Outcomes Study findings and the DUKE profiling method.[3] Ratings of satisfaction or self-examination responses remain difficult to systematically incorporate into physician profiles.[27,28]

With the exception of disease-specific efforts (for instance, diabetes and CHF), the notion of severity ratings based on medical criteria for cross-environment comparisons of sub-populations has not been vigorously pursued. Now, however, the growing transformation to managed care is providing impetus for holistic examination of care processes, and, by implication, is requiring that severity ranking occur outside (i.e., prior to) hospitalization. Models that categorize patients into groups that may be systematically analyzed across care environments now are in beta stages or recently released from beta testing. These models use an episode of care approach in an attempt to link all services associated with a patient's illness.

At this time, models exist that can link illness-specific and wellness services across outpatient-inpatient lines. The ability of current models to link outpatient drug information is weak in most of these models but is being actively pursued. The ability to incorporate laboratory information resulting from decisions in the outpatient world appears to be on the horizon.

Weaknesses in Existing Models

Existing severity-adjustment models suffer from human error and data integrity problems, in addition to gaps in datasets and more technical weaknesses. Iezzoni[29] and Hornbrook *et al.*[30] provide excellent descriptions of the types of shortcomings often encountered in today's adjustment/grouping systems. Three areas will need further attention if a successful adjustment model is to be created.

■ Grouping constructs.

■ Managing medical complications.

■ Handling accounting problems.

Grouping Constructs

How to aggregate the units of analysis, whether the unit of analysis is the patient, the diagnosis code, the illness, or the disease, is the *aggregation problem*. Some models attempt to keep patients whole and adjust for differences in individuals or groups. These models can take into account demographic factors such as race, educational level, age, and sex when grouping individuals in disease groups. DRGs incorporate some of these variables in reimbursement calculations. The CSI system attempts to attach such things as the response rate to therapy and dependency on hospital staff, but it still groups by patient. Other systems, such as DECs and ETGs, attempt to dissect patient data into isolated cost and treatment categories within a particular illness or disease. A patient may be associated with more than one group as a result of this dissecting, but the cost associated with each illness is captured.

FIGURE 2. COMPETING METHODOLOGIES CONTRASTED

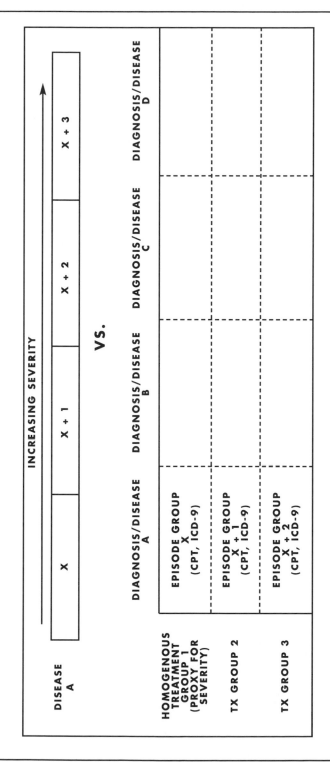

The upper portion depicts a single disease, i.e., diabetes, with increasing severity due to increasing complications and contrasts in the lower section a matrix approach showing grouped treatment patterns for specific disease entities.

FIGURE 3. EPISODE LOGICS

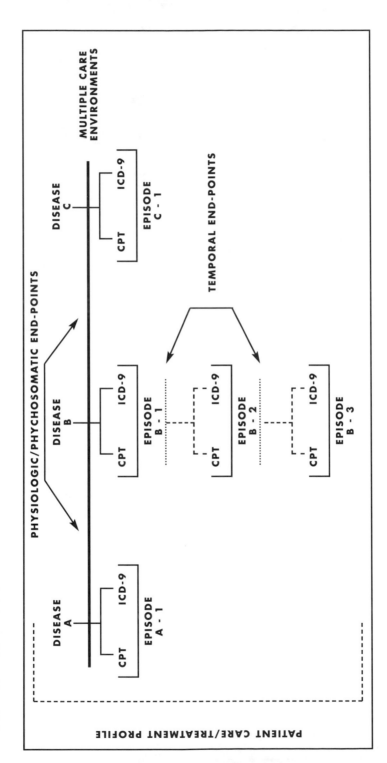

On the other hand, the interactive effects of multiple illnesses in a patient may not be adequately addressed. The Disease Staging approach categorizes information on the basis of the level of disease progression (via related manifestations) in a given patient.

A second grouping problem may be termed the *disaggregation problem.* It reflects the fact that there are disagreements about how to dissect patient data, given that patient information is not going to be examined as a singular unit of analysis. There are two dominant approaches to the disaggregation process. One approach applies a score to each patient according to the level of disease progression. Each of these sub-categories can be used for comparisons of resource intensity, evaluations of physician decision making, etc. The fundamental delineation process is in the level of disease progression, with each level indicating a particular severity. The second approach is to use the types of treatment or treatment/resource intensity as a proxy for severity (figure 2, page 113). Patients may be placed in one or more categories according to the diagnoses (diseases) that are present and the types of treatments provided. These categories may then be compared with expected expenditure/intensity numbers for that area of the matrix.

Managing Medical Complications

The second underlying phenomenon that influences the consistency of severity adjustment across models is the ability of each model to control for medical complications (figure 3, page 114).

On one level, this refers to the ability to distinguish between diseases and multiple occurrences of the same disease. The more sophisticated models distinguish between diseases based on physiological breaking points, and between occurrences of the same diseases based on expected/logical temporal end-points (time span of illness) or clean periods (absence of requests for treatment).

On a more detailed level, however, managing complications implies the ability to control for the additive, interactive, adverse and perverse effects of complications and comorbidities in healing and treatment processes. The inability to control for specific types of complications when developing episode groups affects the reliability and accuracy of both the grouping constructs and the analyses for which they are used.

The manner in which complications are considered varies across models. Horn determined that groups should be categorized by the absence or the existence of a major surgical procedure and that more homogeneous groupings could be determined through examination of interactions, comorbidities, and response to treatment.[31] Iezzoni *et al.* identified 27 potentially preventable in-house

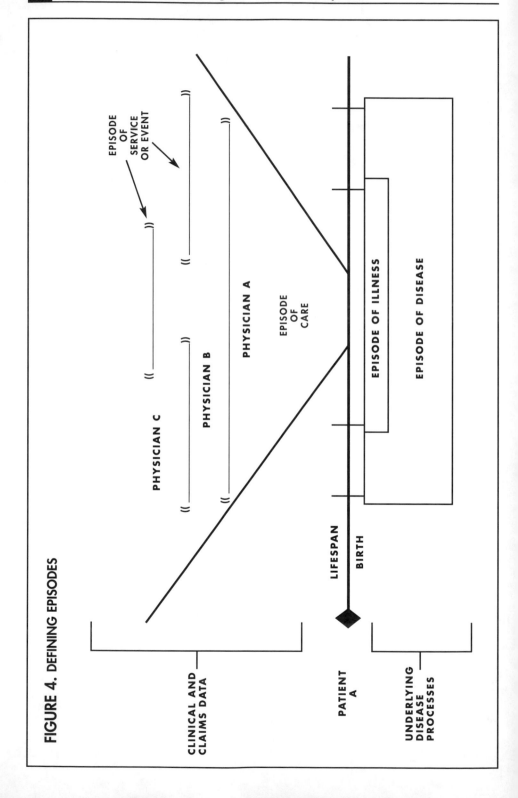

FIGURE 4. DEFINING EPISODES

complications of medical and surgical care.[29] New methodologies may use the comorbidity classification methodology (quantitative index by condition) developed by Charlson *et al.*[32]

Most models, however, continue to suffer from problems identified as early as Hornbrook *et al.*[30] They discussed the need to distinguish between comorbidities caused by environmental factors, by the disease process, and by clinicians, or those that develop during treatment. They presented the need to integrate temporal or physiological end-points that separate repeated acute cases of the same disease, to avoid double or triple counting. In addition, they discussed the importance of developing means by which acute flare-ups of a chronic disease and acute complications of a chronic disease may be identified. To date, grouping/adjustment models have not been developed to adequately address these shortcomings.

Accounting Problems

In addition to design and construct issues, there are accumulation or accounting phenomena that help explain differences in the consistency and reliability of alternative severity-adjustment models. Almost all of the models have been tested using claims data or hospital records. As a result, they are subject to differences in using cost versus billed versus paid dollar amounts when accounting for intra- and extra-class grouping variances. The fact that cost-charge ratios change over time and are not uniform across regions has adverse implications on the accuracy and consistency of model results. The dependent variable of most models also depends on the accuracy and specificity of hospital/claims accounting systems in allocating dollar expenditures/charges to specific departments and services.

Additional accounting problems result from the fact that human error will undoubtedly increase as the opportunity increases for interpretation and hands-on manipulation of data. Data gathered in one place and analyzed in another (i.e., the clinic and the claims department) frequently require re-entry or human-driven data interfacing. The opportunity for errors will expand as the quantity of datasets to be integrated grows. Without automation (i.e., bar coding), the number of errors in a dataset also may be expected to increase as the data-entry quantity and frequency increases over multiple environments.

Accounting problems are also associated with accumulation of medical information. For instance, models (excluding extreme cases that are physiologically driven) generally do not incorporate test results. The primary diagnosis and procedures are used to dissect patient data and to develop expected cost streams. This process ignores the fact that whether any given laboratory test is positive or negative may have significant implications for the cost of treating a disease. (This, of course, is only true if the test would not indicate a disease progression or manifestation that can be captured through a movement from one severity level to another.) Moreover, in certain cases, the response value to a test may have cost, treatment, and/or disease severity implications not accounted for in the constructs of existing models.

Another problem with current accumulation methodology is that medical information extracted from claims databases can imply that information is rolled up to the diagnosis level. All services (and attached charges) that accompany a physician-prescribed diagnosis are attributed to that diagnosis. Whether a particular service is for the prescribed primary diagnosis or some other ailment, the charges still are attributed to the physician assignment. This roll-up of unrelated procedures into a given diagnosis reduces the accuracy of all cost-based models.

The Future of Grouping/Severity of Illness Adjustment Models
Defining Episodes of Care

During the course of pathophysiologic progression, a disease will affect patients differently at different points in time. Patients may have periods of wellness, between which they suffer from diseases in three stages.

The first stage reflects the fact that a disease may affect the health of an individual without his or her knowledge. Further, the disease may affect health before, during, and after medical treatment is provided. In the simplest terms, a disease is present until it no longer is present, as determined by the same (or for that matter improved) tests/criteria that identified its presence. In figure 4, page 116, the episode of disease in a patient's lifespan is represented by the longest bracket.

The second stage of disease reflects the fact that, as progression occurs, an individual eventually will realize something is wrong. This realization is termed an "illness" and represents the ill feeling an individual experiences during this stage. The illness stage can occur only after a disease is present and will occur only as long as a disease is present (but often for a lesser period if treatment is provided). An episode of illness is therefore presented in figure 4 by a subbracket within the "episode of disease" bracket.

The third stage of disease represents abatement, recidivism, or remission during the course of treatment. This stage reflects the fact that weaknesses in physiological or psychological processes often cause individuals to seek professional treatment of an illness. The third stage may include multiple short periods of treatment (i.e., multiple office visits to a provider or visits to referral providers), one long treatment period (i.e., surgery or other inpatient stay), or any other treatment combination. Generally, it is expected that treatment will be for a specific period (antibiotic prescription for 10 days, five physical therapy sessions, etc.) that is shorter than either the period of illness or the disease presence.

This framework creates multiple dilemmas for existing grouping mechanisms. First, episodes of care must remain conceptually and analytically separate from the episode of illness. This is true because different individuals will be more or less sensitive to the pathophysiological processes of the disease. In addition, the episode of care should not be mistaken for the episode of disease. The end-point of an episode of disease can be determined using laboratory/pathology tests, but the beginning may not be known. With certain exceptions for disease-specific, ICU, and inpatient models, existing adjustment mechanisms do not incorporate the level of detail required for such separations. Instead, the grouping of data and severity adjustment occur around a primary diagnosis, and procedures are recorded as part of the billing process. As a result, the quality of severity adjustment must be questioned. For example, two individuals going to the same or different physicians may be attributed with the same diagnosis and procedures, despite the fact that one is more severely ill-has greater physiologic impairment-and may need additional medical care in the future.

Second, allocation to severity groups is based on accumulation of prescribed diagnoses (and/or their additive effects) that cross clinic and care environment boundaries. If this information is not routinely gathered and integrated in its *entirety*, the ascribed severity may be inaccurate. This occurs when analysts, administrators, and/or physicians mistakenly assume that known episodes of service equal an episode of care. This is only true when all services provided for a particular condition are known and all services provided are for the same purpose. Any causes of missing diagnosis codes (i.e., visits outside of a network, fee-for-service visits, or diagnoses attributed under previous insurance plans) pose additional questions about the suitability of adjustments based on globally recorded information.

Third, existing systems ascribe severity from different centrist perspectives using previously collected information. The DEC approach frequently requires up to a year for a particular episode to be considered complete. The ETG approach uses clean periods and therefore does not take into account services sought elsewhere and not captured. In nearly all other approaches as well, the severity of any given patient is retroactively prescribed and is not based on the true physiologic condition at the time of visit. As a result, the severity allocation process is of little practical usefulness to the physician during the course of treatment. Moreover, the information lag to physicians resulting from existing methodologies further reduces the ability of analytical systems to improve operational effectiveness.

The authors believe that a large component in the future development of grouping models will be to increase the ability to extract and provide information to physicians at the point of service. This will require the development of finer delineations of tracked data, and severity within disease, on the basis of a combination of symptoms and laboratory or pathology results.

Linking Episodes of Care

The importance of controlling for the existence of comorbidities has been discussed above. However, the need to identify the interactive and additive effects of more than one illness/disease on patients and populations will be crucial to profiling physicians and managing diseases well into the next decade. The need to identify these effects is hindered by the fact that existing models use a point system based on the existence of another diagnosis; group or flag individuals on the basis of existence of another diagnosis; or, in the extreme, attempt to categorize co-morbidities to account for them.

This process is affected by the same shortcomings of grouping on the basis of diagnosis codes described above. In addition, the fact that more than one diagnosis is being examined creates additional inaccuracies. One of the two or more codes may be recorded for the purpose of ruling out or noting past diagnoses as no longer relevant. This implies that only certain diagnostic, evaluative, or administrative procedures should be allocated to such diagnoses, while the remaining therapeutic services should be applied only to the existing illness.

Additional problems occur when different diagnoses are ascribed by two different physicians or when any physician reverses a diagnosis. In the former situation, time is sometimes used as a proxy for accuracy. The latest diagnosis is considered separately or (if related) is considered the most accurate-without any supporting physiologic evidence by which the conflict may be accurately resolved. When a physician reverses a diagnosis, there is seldom an automated means to determine whether past services should be attributed to the new diagnosis or whether (because of an increase in severity or movement to another group) only services after the new diagnosis should be considered.

As the level of detail of medical information is improved through the introduction of electronic medical records, many of the problems associated with multiple diagnoses will be alleviated. Nonetheless, the ability to evaluate the treatment decisions of physicians will still depend on identification and quantification of disease interactions. On some occasions, we can expect that multiple diagnoses actually will serve to reduce the need for treatment (or will reduce treatment costs over separate occurrences of two diseases). At other times, multiple diagnoses may serve to dramatically increase the amount of services (and costs) associated with effective treatment. In either case, diagnosis codes will

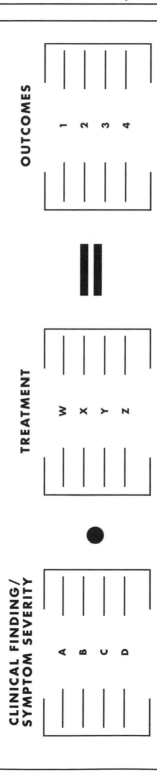

FIGURE 5. DISEASE TREATMENT - OUTCOME RELATIONSHIP

not be sufficient to determine the true impact of multiple diagnoses. Instead, objectively measured physiologic phenomena need to be tracked and associated with treatment decisions.

Using the diagram in figure 5, page 121, it is possible to understand the placement of a number of developments. If tracked information is dissected to the level of signs and symptoms, it will be possible to determine the impact of underlying interactions between pathology and treatment on the health and welfare of individuals. If signs and symptoms are captured and associated with treatment decisions, it will be possible to identify the effect of alternative treatments on outcomes for any given set of conditions. Holding each set of physiological findings and symptoms constant, it will be possible to determine the cost stream and benefits that may be attributed to particular treatment decisions. In this manner, an economic "maximin" solution (maximum benefit attained using the minimum amount of resources necessary) may be achieved. In addition, a preferred method of treatment-likely derived using decision support tools and real data-may be determined for sets of symptoms, rather than subjective assignment of a diagnosis.

Similarly, using this approach, it will be possible to evaluate the effectiveness of existing algorithms for different sets of symptoms. Using existing protocols for treatment (or simply holding constant any treatment component), it will be possible to identify the effect that changes in physiologic conditions have on outcomes and cost. This framework should facilitate the discovery of symptom-treatment connections that cross existing beliefs about disease boundaries, because it does not require that a disease framework is *a priori* identified.

Statistical theory necessitates large databases, if the fine delineations of this approach are to be used for decision-making. Testing for significant between-group differences in outcomes will require that a sufficient number of individuals are tracked within each disease set or treatment set to identify potential improvements to current practices. This is particularly true when one considers that demographic variables such as age, gender, and race will need to be controlled during the population discrimination process. With sufficiently large databases, however, it will be possible to extend the framework to include additional demographic variables, such as the type of employment, educational level, personal risk factors (i.e., smoking and drinking), and marital status.

Linking Care Environments
The charts of figure 6, page 123, present side-by-side comparisons of treatment costs per patient, after adjusting for severity. A profile of physician decision

FIGURE 6

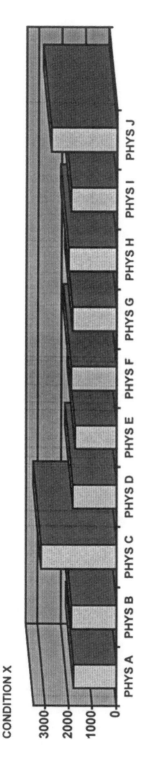

INPATIENT COST PROFILE
BY PHYSICIAN

$ PER PATIENT
CONDITION X

3000 —
2000 —
1000 —
0 —

PHYS A PHYS B PHYS C PHYS D PHYS E PHYS F PHYS G PHYS H PHYS I PHYS J

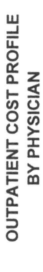

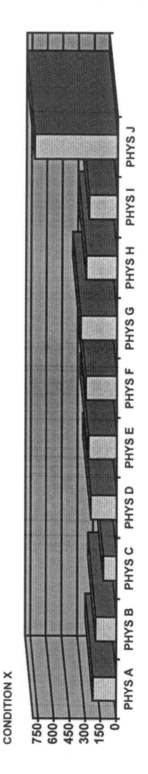

OUTPATIENT COST PROFILE
BY PHYSICIAN

$ PER PATIENT
CONDITION X

750 —
600 —
450 —
300 —
150 —
0 —

PHYS A PHYS B PHYS C PHYS D PHYS E PHYS F PHYS G PHYS H PHYS I PHYS J

making in the inpatient world would lead to the conclusion that Physician C and Physician J are providing more costly care to their patients than is the norm. Conversely, a profile from the outpatient perspective would indicate that Physician C is a very efficient provider of medical services, while Physician J still provides more costly services to patients. A profile of prescription characteristics or referral patterns may yield different conclusions. Relating these input profiles to measures of output (outcomes) may yield further significant changes in the ranking of physicians.

If patients are profiled within single-care environments, the real economic impact of decision making is distorted. Today, this frequently leads to conflicting, misunderstood, or unactionable reports to physicians. It also reduces the ability and credibility of those trying to effectively allocate medical resources.

Note that using more sophisticated presentations, incorporating z-scores or significant differences (t-tests or chi-squares), will not circumvent the problem currently addressed. Only through integration of information across care environments will it be possible to evaluate the treatment decisions of physicians. This is true because treatment decisions made in one setting will affect the treatment outcomes from a different setting. It also is true because the costs attributable to physician decisions cross multiple care environments. Hence decisions in all settings need to be related to outcomes, in order to fairly evaluate physician performance and understand interactions between treatment and pathological processes. Integration of electronic medical records will facilitate medical research efforts, but evaluations also will require integration of financial information from multiple sources.

A serious debate has not yet begun between the users/developers of multiple environment-specific modeling tools and the users/developers of cross-environment modeling tools. The authors believe this future debate will revolve around the accuracy of defining groups that cross care environments versus environment-specific groupings and the predictive accuracy of multiple single-environment models versus the predictive accuracy of any given multi-environment model.

Initially, single-environment tools are likely to make a better showing in both coefficient of variation and explanation of variance (R-squared) terms. However, the trend toward managed care will force greater concentration on the development of cross-environment tracking and evaluation tools. Beginning with further delineations of uniform outpatient-inpatient groupings along staging and episode lines, cross-environment models should develop predictive power equal to or greater than that of multiple single-environment models.

The current debate within cross-care environment modeling revolves around the issue of whether patients should be tracked (and physicians evaluated) on the basis of physiologic severity or homogeneity of treatment. However, both of these concepts still are based on subjective ascription of diagnosis and procedure codes.

In time, a devolution to symptoms will transcend existing disagreements about the basis of categorizing patients. This devolution will facilitate direct integration of information between care environments, because crosswalks between multiple scales or indexes will not need to be developed. Data may then be examined directly through the use of uniform single/composite physiological factors that are objectively determined.

Refining Severity Adjustment

Severity-adjustment mechanisms that have evolved over the past 20 years predominantly use the following premise: Severity and risk can generally be taken as equivalent, and in specific cases may be equated, if we define severity as the risk of loss of physical function.

Despite the mathematical manageability inherent in defining risk/severity in this way, the authors argue against this premise. Disease or illness severity is a physiological condition exhibited through the existence, combination, and intensity of symptoms in any given patient. Risk, on the other hand, is an actuarial probability of a specific outcome. The difference is subtle, but the authors believe it is important.

The calculation of risk requires that a "sufficient number" of "sufficiently similar" individuals have experienced outcomes of particular treatments. If either the treatment or a symptom is new (just discovered or made measurable), calculation of risk-the probability of a specific outcome-is not possible, or is at least highly inaccurate. Alternatively, the discovery of a new treatment or symptom does not hinder identification of severity. Examination of the impact of biological phenomena and their intensity on organs/systems can be identified, at the least, at an atomic level, and related to the effects of alternative treatments or patient groups. Thus, before calculation of risk is possible (because outcomes may not be known), it is possible to apply medically based objective measurements of severity.

Why is this distinction important?

First, science and technology are redefining our understanding of biological organisms and the interaction of these organisms with physiologic growth, aging, and disease transfer. A large body of our future understanding of disease-patient severity and temporal relationships will be based on knowledge gained from genetic sequences. If these genetic sequences are incorporated as definitive control variables in analyses of severity, the accuracy of treatment can be increased and the use of medical/biological indications of severity can be used as feedback into efforts for genomic medicine.

Second, if we move to quantified symptoms or patient-reported functional levels or preferences (not diseases, diagnoses, procedures, etc.) as indicators of severity, it will be possible to create the physiologic equivalent to econometric modeling. Severity can be calculated on an individual basis and associated with a preferred treatment approach.

Integrating Treatment Algorithms

Integrating algorithms into severity-adjustment models should allow for the development of three organizational processes:

■ The ability to relate fine delineations of inputs to fine delineations of outputs.

■ The ability to evaluate actual treatment practices for homogeneous groups.

■ The ability to provide a tool that can be used by physicians at the point of service.

As outlined above, integrating treatment protocols would provide the ability to relate fine delineations of inputs (i.e., medical services and costs) to fine delineations of outputs (medical/physiological outcomes) for specific homogeneous populations with a fixed set of physiological symptoms.

Integrating treatment protocols would enable the evaluation of actual treatment practices for homogenous groups of patients. This should allow for an evolutionary link (CQI) between discoveries made by analyzing actual practice patterns (which feed back into algorithm constructs) and implementation of more effective desired methods of medical practice (which feed back into actual practice).

Integration of protocols associated with asymptotic conditions should provide a tool that may be used by the physician at the point of service. Using the combination of symptoms a patient exhibits, a physician should be able to access the most effective/desirable treatment practice guideline in an automated fashion.

We propose three general practice protocol relationships: those that meet, do not meet, and approximately meet treatment guidelines. It will be important to distinguish on a symptom-group basis between guidelines that have different levels of sophistication. Models of care will have to distinguish among relationships that:

■ Require only specific services to be provided.

■ Require services to be provided in a specific order.

■ Require certain services to be provided before others, between which additional services may be provided at a physician's discretion.

An example of where service composition needs to be considered is well-care. Drawing blood, administering an injection, checking a patient's eyes, and listening to a patient's heart can be performed in any order. Alternatively, approximately equivalent procedures may be allowed in certain cases to provide for physician discretion (for instance, laboratory test A may be substituted for laboratory test B.)

Where the order of treatment occurrence is important, rank-order relationships in practice need to be identified and related to the protocol order. An example of where the order of treatment is important include excalating procedures involved in womens health. Physicians perform a pap smear before a colposcopy, and a colposcopy before a biopsy. Treatment order may be dictated by financial or clinical criteria.

In some cases, less restrictive criteria can be incorporated to allow the occurrence of additional or alternative procedures, as long as the algorithmic order is maintained for symptom-specific procedures.

The above example of treatment guideline comparisons reflects that certain symptom combinations require that specific procedures be performed over time. As long as a core progression is performed, ancillary services may be performed at the physician's discretion. Note that we are not advocating the use of a singular global statistic to indicate the level of association between different practice algorithms. We are instead proposing identification of specific treatment (procedure) deviations from the preferred treatment algorithm, using an automated process. Moreover, we are proposing that comparisons be made between grouped practice patterns (or specific providers) and the desired algorithm, not between alternative treatment algorithms. Superior algorithms will be derived from cost-outcome and treatment-outcome comparisons of alternative treatment practices using actual data.

The ability to shift at will between practice-protocol relationships and between comparison criteria will be important in developing an evolutionary link between medical discoveries and clinical practice. The development of such a tool will further the ability to perform research by allowing for greater flexibility in the analysis of inputs (treatment accumulation) versus outputs. When this tool is combined with physiologic definitions of severity using finer delineations of data than the contemporary ICD-9 coding system, the ability to develop guidance systems for clinical practices will be realized.

Conclusion

In the preceding review of the various methodological and practical issues surrounding the development of a statistically valid and clinically relevant physician profiling tool, the authors have exposed many ancillary issues attendant to the use of administrative and clinical health services data. The authors also have indicated that the tools that will be the most relevant in the actual mining of the vast data warehouses that are forming within the health care delivery system will need to:

■ Include both clinical and administrative data.

■ Roll-up across all care environments.

■ Include information from patients' symptoms, laboratory and diagnostic testing, and pharmacological data.

■ Index severity using clinically relevant and interpretable schemes.

Tools that meet these requirements will allow the most effective research for outcome care innovation and system financial modeling and management. Tools that also imbed within themselves clinical treatment algorithms and update these algorithms with accumulating data will be useful for clinicians at the point of care, and will become invaluable to health services' research.

Progress in this area will be important to clinicians, administrators and researchers alike. Much development already is under way, although it is almost exclusively being performed under proprietary auspices. The obvious need for standardized and flexible analytical tools within this realm must spur more collaboration among researchers, developers, and the eventual clinical users of this work.

It is through this collaboration and joint development of analytical tools and capabilities that we can best meet the information needs of the health care industry and best treat the patients served by our industry as we move into the coming 21st Century.

References

1. Rawson, H. *Unwritten Laws: The Unofficial Rules of Life As Handed Down by Murphy and Other Sages.* New York, N.Y.: Three Rivers Press, 1998.

2. SAS Institute, Inc., Cary, N.C., http//www.sas.com.

3. Parkerson, G., and others. "Health Status and Severity of Illness as Predictors of Outcomes in Primary Care. *Medical Care* 33(1):53-66, Jan. 1995.

4. Testa, M., and Simonson, D. "Assessment of Quality-of-Life Outcomes." *New England Journal of Medicine* 334(13):835-40, March 28, 1996.

5. Knaus, W., and others. "An Evaluation of Outcome from Intensive Care in Major Medical Centers." *Annals of Internal Medicine* 104(3):410-8, March 1986.

6. Knaus, W., and others. "Apache II: A Severity of Disease Classification System." *Critical Care Medicine* 13(10):818-29, Oct. 1985.

7. Knaus, W., and others. "The Apache III Prognostic System: Risk Prediction of Hospital Mortality for Critically Ill Hospitalized Adults." *Chest* 100(6):1619-36, Dec. 1991.

8. Le Gall, J., and others. "A New Simplified Acute Physiology Score (SAPS II) Based on a European/North American Multicenter Study." *JAMA* 270(24):2957-63, March 22, 1993.

9. Lemeshow, S., and Le Gall, J. "Modeling the Severity of Illness of ICU Patients: A System Update." *JAMA* 272(13):1049-55, Oct. 5, 1994.

10. Lemeshow, S., and others. "Mortality Probability Models for Patients in the Intensive Care Unit for 48 or 72 Hours: A Prospective Multicenter Study." *Critical Care Medicine* 22(9):1351-8, Sept. 1994.

11. Lemeshow, S., and others. "Refining Intensive Care Unit Outcome Prediction by Using Changing Probabilities of Mortality." *Critical Care Medicine* 16(5):470-7, May 1998.

12. Lemeshow, S., and others. "Mortality Probability Models (MPM II) Based on an International Cohort of Intensive Care Unit Patients." *JAMA* 270(20):2478-86, Nov. 24, 1993.

13. Fery-Lemonnier, E., and others. "Evaluation of Severity Scoring Systems in ICUs-Translation, Conversion, and Definition Ambiguities as a Source of Inter-Observer Variability in Apache II, SAPS, and OSF." *Intensive Care Medicine* 21(4):356-60, April 1995.

14. Horn, S., and others. "The Relationship between Severity of Illness and Hospital Length of Stay and Mortality." *Medical Care* 29(4):305-17, April 1991.

15. Horn, S., and Horn, R. "The Computerized Severity Index: A New Tool for Case-Mix Management." *Journal of Medical Systems* 10(1):73-8, Feb. 1986.

16. Cave, D. "Analyzing the Content of Physicians' Medical Practices." *Journal of Ambulatory Care Management* 17(3):15-36, July 1994.

17. Cave, D., and Geehr, E. "Analyzing Patterns of Treatment Data to Provide Feedback to Physicians." *Medical Interface* 7(7):117-26,128, July 1994.

18. Cave, D. "Pattern-of-Treatment Differences among Primary Care Physicians in Alternative Systems of Care." *Benefits Quarterly* 10(3):6-19, Third Quarter 1994.

19. Cave, D. "Profiling Physician Practice Patterns Using Diagnostic Episode Clusters." *Medical Care* 33(5):463-86, May 1995.

20. Dang, D., and others. "Episode Treatment Groups: An Illness Classification and Episode Building System-Part II." *Medical Interface* 9(4):122-8, April 1996.

21. Knaus, W., and others. "Variations in Mortality and Length of Stay in Intensive Care Units." *Annals of Internal Medicine* 118(10):753-61, May 15, 1993.

22. Young, W., and others. "PMC Patient Severity Scale: Derivation and Validation." *Health Services Research* 29(3):367-90, Aug. 1994

23. Thomas, J.and Ashcraft, M. "Measuring Severity of Illness: Six Severity Systems and Their Ability to Explain Cost Variations." *Inquiry* 28(1):39-55, Spring 1991.

24. Iezzoni, L., and others. "Admission Medisgroups Score and the Cost of Hospitalizations." *Medical Care* 26(11):1068-80, Nov. 1988.

25. Tierney, W., and others. "Predicting Inpatient Costs with Admitting Clinical Data." *Medical Care* 33(1):1-14, Jan. 1995.

26. Iezzoni, L., and others. "Admission and Mid-Stay Medisgroups Scores as Predictors of Hospitalization Charges." *Medical Care* 29(3):210-20, March 1991.

27. Katz, J., and others. "Can Comorbidity Be Measured by Questionnaire Rather Than Medical Record Review?" *Medical Care* 34(1):73-84, Jan. 1996.

28. Mancuso, C., and Charlson, M. "Does Recollection Error Threaten the Validity of Cross-Sectional Studies of Effectiveness." *Medical Care* 33(4 Suppl.):AS77-88, April 1995.

29. Iezzoni, L., and others. "Identifying Complications of Care Using Administrative Data." *Medical Care* 32(7):700-15, July 1994.

30. Hornbrook, M., and others. "Health Care Episodes: Definition, Measurement, and Use." *Medical Care Review* 42(2):163-218, Fall 1985.

31. Horn, S., and others. "Measuring Severity of Illness: Homogeneous Case Mix Groups." *Medical Care* 21(1):14-30, Jan. 1983.

32. Charlson, M., and others. "A New Method of Classifying Prognostic Comorbidity in Longitudinal Studies: Development and Validation." *Journal of Chronic Diseases* 40(5):373-83, 1987.

David M. Klubert, MD, is Chief Knowledge Officer and Colt G. Courtright, MPA, is Senior Scientist, Ruffin Informatics, Inc., Portland, Oregon.

SECTION III

Physician Profiling in Practice

CHAPTER 8

Hospital Physician Profiling:
Education-Based Practice Pattern Analysis
by Frederic G. Jones, MD, CPE, FACPE, and
Craig C. Johnson, MHA, MPH

*I*n 1993, the authors published a case study on a data-driven and education-based approach to practice analysis in the hospital setting.[1] This system was developed in 1988 and has continued in use at Anderson Area Medical Center, a 500-bed community teaching hospital in Anderson, South Carolina. Since the initial report, the process has continued to be refined and is the subject of this report. A recent guide to provider practice profiling[2] suggested that such performance profiling might prove to be a panacea for managing the use and the cost of health care. In that context, data about cost, frequency, and quality of health care services are translated into information to be used in improvement activities. The article made several key points that we will comment on and share our personal experiences. It is important to note that much of the current literature pertains to the managed care model, with economic profiling as a major goal.

"Buy-in" by practitioners to the purposes and the methodology of a profiling system is key to initial acceptance and continued support of the system's processes. A case-mix-adjusted approach is essential to reassure those being assessed that consideration of their patient population has not been neglected. From the outset, a physician advisory group has been active in guiding hospital administration in the process. The vice president for medical affairs (VPMA) has played a key role in the development of the process, assisted by the hospital's full-time informaticist, the clinical performance department (formerly QA and UR), and a university statistician, in a consulting role. More recently, an RN, PhD, with a strong case management background,. has become a key member of this team. This has enabled multidisciplinary teams to incorporate evidence-based guidelines into plans of care. Analyses of the work of these teams have become a key component of the periodic reports provided to individual practitioners. Finally, the VPMA has also occupied the position of Director of Medical Education. In that capacity, he has scheduled 50-60 accredited CME hours per year with close coordination to findings of the profiling studies. Furthermore, a family medicine residency program affiliated with the hospital has afforded faculty and voluntary attending physicians the opportunity to introduce future practitioners to these concepts of feedback and improvement.

One should certainly ask if there is evidence that improvement has occurred as a result of this methodology and its associated hospitalwide activities. We have been fortunate to present these data on a number of occasions at national meetings and have had a number of reviewers address these efforts The most recent reviewer was Michael Millenson, author of *Demanding Medical Excellence*[3] and nominee for the Pulitzer Prize for his five-part series on medical quality issues in the *Chicago Tribune* in 1993. Likewise, Dr. Michael Pine, who often writes of important considerations in physician profiling,[4] has periodically reviewed the results of our work for a number of years. In 1992, the medical center embraced the Deming approach to continuous quality improvement as a core strategy and incorporated the principles advocated by Berwick and Nolan.[5] A further outgrowth of the Anderson profiling effort was the development of a patient-level indicator monitoring system that was ultimately utilized by some 40 South Carolina hospitals and approved by the Joint Commission on Accreditation of Healthcare Organizations in its ORYX project.

We have learned that frequent feedback is key to sustaining improvement and revisit studied medical conditions and procedures at intervals of no more than 18 months. This approach has resulted in prioritization of our efforts so that the hospital administration and the medical staff agree on issues that warrant these rather intense efforts. Naturally, a study can be initiated on the basis of findings of clinical performance activities or at the request of medical staff departments and committees or of the plan of care teams. Close collaboration with the South Carolina Professional Review Organization also leads to topic selection. On occasions, an individual practitioner requests a study and, when possible, this request is honored. More often, as a result of the confidential performance report provided, the physician will request additional information on how his or her performance compares with that of a peer group. The hospital has a comprehensive cost accounting system that allows one to "drill down" for such detail. In addition, the medical center participates in a number of regional and national databases and benchmarking efforts. The National Registry for Myocardial Infarction is one that has been particularly helpful.

We are not reluctant to incorporate approaches used by others in the field. Brent James, MD, is a pioneer of physician profiling and likes to tell people how sharing data with physicians can transform and improve the way in which they practice medicine. The goal of profiling, Dr. James says, is to identify variables-what physicians do differently-and then to try to understand and learn from the reasons behind their decisions. James' colleagues at Intermountain Health Care reported on critical factors in reducing post-operative wound infections.[6] This led to the development of an improvement team that has monitored performance and provided regular feedback to all who perform procedures at our facility.

An editorial on the use and abuse of practice profiles[7] suggested that, in 1994, none of the profiles in use were adequate to the task. One would hope that methodologies have continued to evolve and justify this latest form of practitioner oversight. Richard Thompson, MD, who suggested the current model for quality oversight and accountability at Anderson in 1980, has recently written on the topic now and in the future."[8] His article explores a plan on how to proceed with evaluating physician performance. In addition, David Nash, MD, has recently issued a "Report on Report Cards."[9] In his analysis, there appears to be convincing evidence that, at the system level, report cards stimulate change in the right direction. Dr. Nash conducted grand rounds at Anderson in the early 1990s. In earlier years, officials from organized medicine were both anxious and skeptical about the value of profiling. In a recent JAMA policy perspectives,[10] that point of view appears to have moderated. More recently, A JAMA article reports on the unreliability of individual physician "report cards" in diabetes care.[11] The accompanying editorial asks, "Can Physician Profiles Be Trusted."[12] Letters responding to these articles constitute a basis for weighting the advantages and disadvantages of the approach.[13] There appears to be general agreement that improving the quality of health care is a desirable goal by improving one or more elements of Donabedian's triad of structure, process, and outcome.

Epstein likens such reporting to the Wright brothers' early airplane, now rolling down the runway. If we are patient and persistent, he says, quality reporting could take us aloft.[10]

At Anderson Area Medical Center, we have been encouraged by the strong support for this endeavor. In this era of accountability, predicted by Relman,[14] health care professionals must strive to allay the public's apprehension about cost and quality of the services we provide. It is our belief that practice pattern analysis offers a formidable tool in ensuring that our citizens receive value in their encounters with the health care system.[15]

An example of the AAMC approach to physician profiling is shown in the following case for acute myocardial infarction (AMI). Each physician who cares for AMI patients would receive a similar document, comparing his or her performance with that of other physicians in both a prose report and in tabular form. AMI is only one of many conditions that can be selected for this treatment. In earlier HCFA hospital mortality reports, our hospital was a high-mortality facility. These and other efforts resulted in a 50 percent reduction in mortality for AMI over five years compared with a national reduction of less than 15 percent.

Conclusion:

With our educational approach to physician practice analysis, we strive to take complex data and present them in a simplified form that permits busy physicians to quickly assimilate information. Physicians with the interest and time can explore the variability of several practice parameters among their peers. The final pages of 6-12 Pareto charts are perhaps most important. Physicians can instantly determine if they are above or below the group mean for any given parameter of practice, if they are an outlier. individual physician values are highlighted in fluorescent color allowing instant access to personal values. Physician names are blinded and physician codes are randomized with every report to preserve confidentiality.

Physicians are best qualified to evaluate clinical practice. The ultimate measure of success for our methodology has been to have members of the medical staff request medical records for personal review after having received our practice pattern reports.

Our experience strongly supports the view that educational approaches can be effective in producing practice changes and improved clinical outcomes without telling staff members how to practice medicine. We have seen heartening changes in clinical outcomes at the same time we have seen substantial reductions in the consumption of hospital resources.[16-18] Educational approaches to practice pattern evaluation can be as effective as reports generated for "economic credentialing" and at the same time can preserve medical staff/hospital relationships.

References

1. Jones, F. "Education-Based Practice Pattern Analysis: A Tool for Continuous Improvement of Patient Care Quality." *American Journal of Medical Quality* 7(4):120-4, Winter 1992.

2. Balas, E., and others. "Effect of Physician Profiling on Utilization: Meta-Analysis of Randomized Clinical Trials." *Journal of General Internal Medicine* 11(10):584-90, Oct. 1996.

3. Millenson, M. *Demanding Medical Excellence: Doctors and Accountability in the Information Age.* Chicago, Ill.: University of Chicago Press, 1997.

4. Balsamo, R., and Pine, M. "Important Considerations in Using Indicators to Profile Physicians." *Physician Executive* 21(5):38-45, May 1995.

5. Berwick, D., and Nolan, T. "Physicians as Leaders in Improving Health Care: A New Series in Annals of Internal Medicine." *Annals of Internal Medicine* 128(4):289-92, Feb. 15, 1998.

6. Cross, M. "All for One, One for All." *Modern Physician* 2(5):50-4, May 1998.

7. Kassirer, J. "The Use and Abuse of Practice Profiles." *New England Journal of Medicine* 330(9):634-6, March 3, 1994.

8. Thompson, R. "Physician Report Cards." *Physician Executive* 24(1):46-50, Jan.-Feb. 1998.

9. Nash, D. "Report on Report Cards." *Health Policy Newsletter* 11(2):1-2, May 1998.

10. Epstein, A. "Rolling Down the Runway: The Challenges Ahead for Quality Report Cards." *JAMA* 279(21):1691-6, June 3, 1998

11. Hofer, T., and others. "The Unreliability of Individual Physician 'Report Cards' for Assessing the Costs and Quality of Care of a Chronic Disease." *JAMA* 281(22):2098-105, June 9, 1999.

12. Bindman, A. "Can Physician Profiles Be Trusted?" *JAMA* 281(22):2142-3, June 9, 1999.

13. Letters. *JAMA* 283(1); 41-4, Jan. 5, 2000.

14. Relman, A. "Assessment and Accountability—The Third Revolution in Medical Care." *New England Journal of Medicine* 319(18):1220-2, Nov. 3, 1998.

15. Jones, F., and Duncan, D. *Regulation in the Era of Accountability: Handbook of Health Policy and Administration.* Monticello, N.Y.: Marcel Dekker, Inc., 1998.

16. Johnson, C., and Martin M. "Effectiveness of a Physician Education Program in Reducing Consumption of Hospital Resources in Elective Total Hip Replacement." *Southern Medical Journal*, March, 1996.

17. Johnson, C., and Martin M. "Lowering Physician Hospital Resource Consumption Using Low-Cost Low-Technology Computing." *Proceedings*, 19th Symposium on Computer Applications in Health Care, Nov. 1995.

18. Jones F., and Johnson, C. "Using Outcome Data to Focus Clinical Process Improvement," *Clinical Outcomes*, Health Sciences Institute, Fall 1993.

19. Jones, F. "An Educational Approach to Physician Involvement." In *Increasing Physician Involvement in Quality Improvement Programs*, E., Geehr and Pine, J., Editors. Tampa, Fla.: American College Physician Executives, 1993.

20. Johnson, C., and others. "The Effect of a Physician Education Program on Hospital Length of Stay and Total Patient Charges." *Journal of the South Carolina Medical Association*, June 1993.

Frederic G. Jones, MD, CPE. FACPE, was formerly Executive Vice President for Medical Affairs at Anderson Area Medical Center, Anderson, S.C.. He is now Medical Director of the Anderson Healthwise Initiative. Craig C. Johnson, MHA, MPH, is Medical Informaticist, Anderson Area Medical Center.

Physician Practice Performance
Individual Physician Summary
Physician #999

Acute Myocardial Infarction

Hospital Summary
Mortality

During Fiscal Years 1995 and 96, there were 790 inpatient admissions for the treatment of acute myocardial infarction (AMI) at Anderson Area Medical Center (AAMC). Overall mortality declined from a high of 19.2 percent in FY1987 to a low of 8.9 percent in FY1992. HCFA (Medicare) 30-day mortality at AAMC dropped from 39 percent to 16.7 percent from FY1987 to FY1990, while national HCFA mortality dropped from 26 percent to 23 percent in the same period. AAMC made most remarkable gains on AMI mortality following a multidisciplinary approach to the management of AMI patients.

Recent (through June 1996) NRMI II (National Registry of Myocardial Infarction) data suggest Anderson Area Medical Center (AAMC) may be experiencing high mortality among its acute myocardial infarction patients. These data indicate state mortality is 12.7 percent and national mortality is 10.5 percent. AAMC mortality was reported as being 15.1 percent.

Treatment

According to NRMI II, nontransfer AAMC patients are receiving thrombolysis 29.6 percent of the time, and all South Carolina patients receive it 31.9 percent of the time, with an additional 6.7 percent receiving alternate reperfusion. Nationally, 27 percent of patients received thrombolytics and 7 percent received other forms of initial reperfusion. Recent findings suggest that, in community hospitals, PTCA and thrombolytics have equal outcomes in terms of mortality. AAMC use of IV beta blockers is 29 percent versus 13 percent for the state. AAMC use of oral beta blockers is 51 percent versus 34 percent for the state. AAMC use of ASA, nitrates, and heparin is equal or greater than state averages. AAMC use of calcium channel blockers is 8 percent versus 19 percent for the state.

The interval between symptom onset and administration of thrombolytic therapy at AAMC was 169 minutes, compared to 145 minutes for the state. This indicates success in community education, as early NRMI data suggested that Anderson county residents waited nearly twice as long as state or national groups to seek treatment. The interval between hospital arrival and administration of thrombolytic therapy (door to needle) is 42 minutes compared to 30 minutes for the state. At AAMC, 15 minutes were used for the interval between decision and drug administration versus 9 minutes for the state.

The literature strongly supports timely use of aspirin, thrombolytics, and beta blockers in the early management of AMI. The use of heparin and nitrates is also beneficial. The use of many of these therapeutic modalities increased in 1996. Calcium channel blockers have not been demonstrated to be helpful and their use dropped appropriately.

Your Summary

Your admissions for AMI in FY1995 and 1996 totaled 29. A comparison of your patients with all other AMI patients admitted to AAMC during these two years is provided below:

	Yours	**HW**
Average Age	65.3 years	66.7 years
% Caucasian	82.8%	86.5%
% Male	72.4%	61.3%

Quality Issues

The mortality rate for your patients was 17.2 percent, compared to your peers' rate of 14.3 percent. Of these deaths, 0.0 percent occurred within two days of admission, the HW rate was 38.1%. The mortality figures are crude rates and therefore would also include patients with a "NO-CODE" status (adjustments for no-code status can be made in the future if data are made available). Your readmission rate within 31 days was 13.8 percent compared to the hospitalwide readmission rate of 8.614 percent. 13.8 percent of your patients had "recorded" hospital-incurred complications (narrowly defined by ICD9 996 to 999), with a hospitalwide rate of 15.6 percent, where Medical Records coded these occurrences. 0.0 percent of your patients had "recorded" hospital-incurred infections, with a hospitalwide rate of 7.6 percent, where Medical Records coded these occurrences.

Resource Utilization and Treatment Issues

Listed below are comparisons between you and your peers for utilization of hospital resources as measured by LOS, per diem charges, and charge ratios. Charge profiles are presented as indicators of your resource utilization. The ancillary/total charge ratio is indicative of treatment intensity, with higher ratios being suggestive of higher treatment intensity. The average # of consults requested per patient is also displayed and is an important issue, because MI patients receiving consults have higher average LOS and total charges than nonconsult patients. In a number of cases, consult patients were sicker and justified greater LOS and resource consumption.

	Yours	Peers
Average LOS (Days)	5.8	6.1
Average Number of Consults	0.62	0.46
Ancillary/Total Charge (Ratio)	0.32	0.40
Per Diem Charges	$ 2,930	$ 2,408
Average Total Charges	$17,056	$14,593
Average Ancillary Charge	$ 5,548	$ 5,896
Average Pharmacy Charges	$ 2,668	$ 2,952
Average Respiratory Charges	$ 608	$ 674
Average Laboratory Charges	$ 1,726	$ 1,745

Recent Study Findings
Treatment Delay

The median time between onset of chest pain and presentation at the ED was 5.3 hours in Anderson County from July 1, 1992, through December 31, 1992. From January 1, 1993, through June 30, 1993, median time dropped to 4 hours. A communitywide education program in February 1993 may have contributed to this reduction. In spite of continued improvement, many patients still fall outside the window of opportunity for thrombolytic therapy. Public education is essential if this delay is to be further reduced. Studies reveal a 1 percent mortality in MI patients to be possible with ideal emergency services and prompt action on the part of the patient at time of pain onset.

Contraindication

There continues to be a hesitation to use thrombolytics on the part of many physicians because of fear of inducing an intra-cranial bleed or because the patient is 75 years of age or more. Age in and of itself is no longer seen as an adequate reason for exclusion from thrombolytic therapy. Use after six hours from pain onset remains equivocal. Some studies suggest benefit accrues when it is given in the 6-12 hour period following pain onset. NRMI demonstrated in 1993 that the group of patients benefiting most from thrombolytic therapy were age 80-85. Several litigations are presently in progress for failure to use thrombolytics.

FIGURE 1. MORTALITY RATE BY PHYSICIAN
(ACUTE MYOCARDIAL INFARCTION)

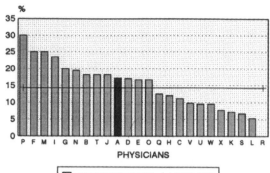

MEDICAL INFORMATICS, 1996

FIGURE 2. COMPLICATION RATE BY PHYSICIAN
(ACUTE MYOCARDIAL INFARCTION)

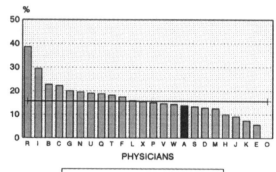

MEDICAL INFORMATICS, 1996

FIGURE 3. NOSOCOMIAL INFECTIONS BY PHYSICIAN
(ACUTE MYOCARDIAL INFARCTION)

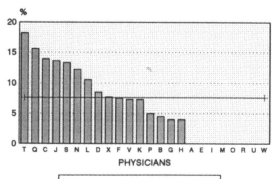

MEDICAL INFORMATICS, 1996

FIGURE 4. AVERAGE LOS (DAYS) BY PHYSICIAN
(ACUTE MYOCARDIAL INFARCTION)

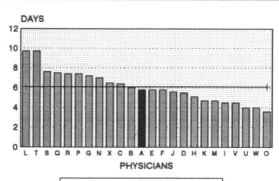

MEDICAL INFORMATICS, 1996

FIGURE 5. AVERAGE TOTAL CHARGES BY PHYSICIAN
(ACUTE MYOCARDIAL INFARCTION)

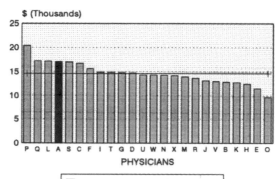

MEDICAL INFORMATICS, 1996

FIGURE 6. READMIT RATE BY PHYSICIAN
(ACUTE MYOCARDIAL INFARCTION)

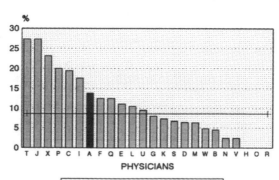

MEDICAL INFORMATICS, 1996

FIGURE 7. PER DIEM CHARGES BY PHYSICIAN
(ACUTE MYOCARDIAL INFARCTION)

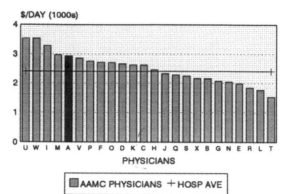

MEDICAL INFORMATICS, 1996

FIGURE 8. CONSULT RATE BY PHYSICIAN
(ACUTE MYOCARDIAL INFARCTION)

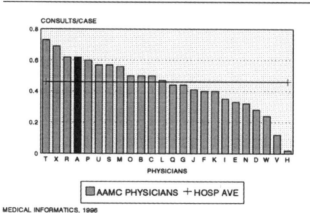

MEDICAL INFORMATICS, 1996

FIGURE 9. CHARGE RATIO BY PHYSICIAN
(ACUTE MYOCARDIAL INFARCTION)

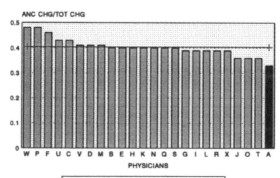

MEDICAL INFORMATICS, 1996

FIGURE 10. CONCOMITANT MEDICATIONS, AMI
(ANDERSON AREA MEDICAL CENTER)

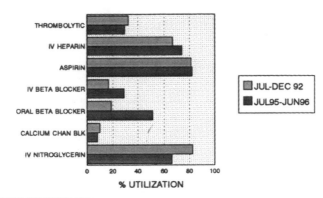

MEDICAL INFORMATICS, 1996

FIGURE 11. USE OF THROMBOLYTICS
(ANDERSON AREA MEDICAL CENTER)

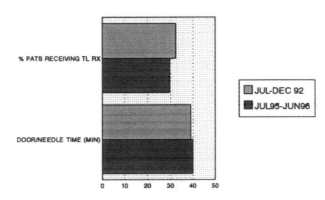

MEDICAL INFORMATICS, 1996

FIGURE 12. USE OF MEDICATIONS WITHIN 24 HOURS
(ANDERSON AREA MEDICAL CENTER)

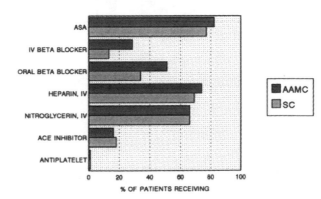

MEDICAL INFORMATICS, 1996

TABLE 1. PHYSICIAN PRACTICE PERFORMANCE

ACUTE MYOCARDIAL INFARCTION

PHYSICIANS	MD CODE	# OF PATIENTS	MORTALITY	READMIT RATE	NOS COMPLICATIONS	NOS INFECTIONS	LOS	AVG TOTAL CHGS	PER DIEM
	A	29	17.2	13.8	13.8	0.0	5.8	$17,075	$2,930
	B	22	18.2	4.5	22.7	4.5	6.0	$12,836	$2,156
	C	36	11.1	19.4	22.2	13.9	6.4	$16,756	$2,622
	D	47	17.0	6.4	12.8	8.5	5.5	$14,749	$2,666
	E	18	16.7	11.1	5.6	0.0	5.8	$11,477	$1,986
	F	40	25.0	12.5	17.5	7.5	5.8	$15,622	$2,717
	G	25	20.0	8.0	20.0	4.0	7.2	$4,799	$2,067
	H	50	12.0	0.0	10.0	4.0	5.1	$12,436	$2,457
	I	17	23.5	17.6	29.4	0.0	4.5	$14,864	$3,281
	J	22	18.2	27.3	9.1	13.6	5.6	$13,124	$2,326
	K	55	7.2	7.3	7.3	7.3	4.7	$12,476	$2,629
	L	19	5.3	10.5	15.8	10.5	9.7	$17,180	$1,764
	M	16	25.0	6.3	1.5	0.0	4.7	$13,933	$2,972
	N	41	19.5	2.4	19.5	12.2	7.0	$14,242	$2,041
	O	18	16.7	0.0	0.0	0.0	3.6	$9,635	$2,709
	P	20	30.0	20.0	15.0	5.0	7.4	$20,404	$2,757
	Q	32	12.5	12.5	18.8	15.6	7.5	$17,241	$2,289
	R	13	0.0	0.0	38.5	0.0	7.4	$13,632	$1,845
	S	30	6.7	6.7	13.3	13.3	7.6	$17,020	$2,249
	T	11	18.2	27.3	18.2	18.2	9.7	$14,850	$1,526
	U	21	9.5	9.5	19.0	0.0	4.0	$14,303	$3,534
	V	41	9.8	2.4	14.6	7.3	4.5	$12,973	$2,860
	W	21	9.5	4.8	14.3	0.0	4.0	$14,287	$3,530
	X	13	7.7	23.1	15.4	7.7	6.5	$14,152	$2,164
	ALL	**790**	**14.3**	**8.6**	**15.6**	**7.6**	**6.1**	**$14,594**	**$2,408**

CHAPTER 9

Medical Group Practice Looks Back on Physician Profiling . . . and Forward

by Angelo P. Spoto Jr., MD, FACP

A story is told of a rich Texan, determined to build a world-class golf course, visiting St. Andrews in Scotland in awe. He sought out the groundskeeper and asked how he might duplicate such a treasure. The man replied, "First you find the perfect picturesque site; you bring in the finest golf architects and site preparers; you purchase the finest grasses; flora, and sands; and you maintain the course with the finest workers, seeds, herbicides, and pesticides. Then you repeat the process for 400 years." This story demonstrates a process not unlike that necessary to develop a high-quality group practice.

Watson Clinic, a limited liability partnership, is a 175-physician multispecialty medical group located in central Florida. Its physicians first started practicing in Lakeland, Florida, in 1914 and became a medical group of five physicians in 1941.[1] Since 1954, it has been a medical partnership, and, since 1995, an LLP. In 1984, certain physicians elected to incorporate their practices. Watson Clinic now operates out of its Lakeland headquarters and 17 regional sites with more than 1,000 employees. Governance is provided by a seven-person Board of Directors (until 1998 called an Executive Committee led by a Managing Partner) elected by the partnership. In 1960, Watson Clinic created the Watson Clinic Foundation, a 501(c)3 foundation involved in medical research, education, and service. A separate, wholly owned entity, the Watson Clinic Center for Research, Inc., was formed in 1985 and carries out research projects involving pharmaceuticals and medical devices. With its creation, all non-basic science research performed by the foundation was transferred to the Center.

The Clinic's primary hospital is Lakeland Regional Medical Center (LRMC), a city-owned, acute care hospital with 851 licensed beds (operating 650) located one block from the Clinic's main campus. Clinic physicians make up 50 percent of the hospital's medical staff.

Although they may not have realized it, physician groups many years ago began profiling physicians in a rudimentary way. The unified medical record allowed physicians in the same specialty or in different specialties to routinely monitor one another's work, albeit in a nonthreatening environment. Watson Clinic in Lakeland, Florida, was no different. It was not uncommon to hear, "Why did you order that calcium on Mrs. Brown?" or "Do you think Cefaclor is the right antibiotic for Mr. Jenkins' bronchitis?" The Clinic's informal profiling has frequently been more important than its formal profiling.

As times changed, and the Clinic's environment changed, Watson Clinic medical care and delivery systems had to change. Increasing complexity has required increasing accountability. Thus evolved formal physician profiling.[2]

Rudimentary economic physician profiling occurred early in previous generations of group practices and was based on various types of office care; hospital care; and, increasingly, both inpatient and outpatient surgeries and procedures. This led to a profiling of fee structures and revenues. Overhead was calculated into the system. In fact, these profiles were worked into cost bases and ultimately into physician compensation distribution formulas. Watson Clinic computerized its billing system in 1962, allowing the computer to analyze patients' accounts and send notices on the basis of how accounts were being handled by patients and their insurance companies. These same computer systems, powerful for the time, were used to profile per physician revenues and to determine physician incomes by a distribution model.

In the mid-1980s, the Clinic and LRMC began to actively discuss quality assurance (QA) and, subsequently, continuous quality improvement (CQI). Although managed care entities had profiled physician allocation of resources for many years, the Clinic minimally documented this allocation, even as owners of a health maintenance organization (HMO), Health Alliance Plan of Florida, from 1985 to 1990. To increase access to the clinic's vast medical information databases, an electronic medical record (EMR) was put into use in 1997.

Profiling the Group Entity

Watson Clinic attempts, by an internal process, to provide for an internal audit and on-site reviews. An active CQI Committee of 10 physicians and administrators was established in 1984 and meets monthly. The committee's major objective is to promote improvement in the quality of patient care through evaluation of data collected through various disease/problem-related studies or projects.

The two major components of Watson Clinic's Quality Improvement Plan involve securing measurements and determining the degree to which standards are met and introducing change based on comparing the information obtained with the goal for improvement. The measurement may be based on structural criteria that focus on the nature of events and activity in the delivery of care or on outcome criteria that describe the result of care or a measurable change in process to improve care or eliminate a problem. Major emphasis now is on outcomes and satisfaction.

In 1994 the Watson Clinic Nephrology Service and Kidney Dialysis Service began participating in a Unit Specific Report (USR) for dialysis patients. It contains Standardized Mortality Ratios (SMRs), Standardized Hospitalization Ratios (SHRs), and Standardized Transplantation Ratios (STRs) for our facility compared to local and national averages. This information allows facilities to evaluate characteristics of patients; patterns of treatment; and patterns of hospitalization, mortality, and transplantation rates with the hope of stimulating internal analysis of quality improvement opportunities and therefore improving the care of the ESRD patient. The Watson Clinic Kidney Center also carries on some 14 QA/ CQI studies pertaining to unit activities.

In 1998, a study of cardiology rehabilitation patients on beta blockers showed a Watson Clinic attainment of 63 percent (national average was 49-51 percent).

There are currently 27 active protocols carried out by six services in an atmosphere of "careful inquisitiveness." by the Clinic's Center for Research. These research protocols are monitored by the Investigational Review Committee of the Center and by the LRMC Institutional Review Board (IRB).

Through the auspices of a federal Health Care Quality Improvement Program (Title X of the Social Security Act), an extensive study of diabetic patients' charts was instituted in 1997 using a state grant. Charts were reviewed for overall quality of care of diabetic patients and converted to indices. The study was repeated in 1998 for comparison purposes. Some improvement was noted in the quality indicators of the study.

A Diabetes HCFA/NCQA/ADA/QI study of 400 patients performed in 1996 was repeated in 1998 using the EMR. Watson Clinic performance was measured against nationally published results using some of 10 measurements, including Hemoglobin-A1C (Hgb A1C). Our frequency of obtaining urinalyses improved 18 percent over the baseline, testing for microalbuminaria increased 42 percent, and prescriptions for ACE inhibitors improved by 41 percent. The results demonstrated a significant improvement in the collaborators as a group, Watson Clinic being one of four in the group.

In 1998, the Watson Clinic Diabetes Education Center instituted a quality diabetes self-management program consisting of comprehensive education and ongoing monitoring, including evaluations of Hgb A1C. The average Hgb A1C fell from 9.8 pre- to 7.2 post-education.

In 1994, a clinicwide survey of anticoagulated patient monitoring was performed. Its findings indicated significant upside improvement potential. After an education program, a repeat study indicated no change. A centralized Coumadin Clinic was planned and instituted. Results were a marked improvement in compliance monitoring capability and therapeutic results. We now follow 2,500 patients in the program.

The Clinic is also involved in "outcomes projects." In 1996, the clinic participated in a standardized patient satisfaction survey. Specialties evaluated included gastroenterology, otolaryngology, cardiology, and general surgery. Watson Clinic results were significantly above national norms.

In June 1998, a clinicwide physician referral satisfaction survey was begun. The intention was to rate satisfaction with departments' inpatient and outpatient care and consultation responsiveness as well as outside referral needs. By August 1999, 48 departments had been evaluated. Results are being tabulated. Three additional studies are to be completed. Their results will be shared with medical administration and the evaluated departments.

In June 1998, in preparation for a possible affiliation with Phy-Cor, Inc., a physician practice management company (PPM), a physician opinion survey was undertaken to compare the feelings and opinions of Watson Clinic physicians with those of physicians in the Phy-Cor data bank. The measurements included practice, administration, and facility satisfaction. Watson Clinic physicians were more satisfied with their practices than the norms. The affiliation discussions did not come to fruition.

Choosing Physicians

The Watson Clinic extensively profiles the individual physician in an attempt to create overall quality for the clinic. If individual quality is sought, expected, evaluated, and maintained, group quality will follow naturally.

The Watson Clinic's early entry into physician profiling included the following:

■ Physicians were required to pass an examination by the Florida State Board of Medical Examiners beginning in 1921.

■ Passing a separate examination by the Board of Examiners in the Basic Sciences became a prerequisite to the Medical Examiners exam in 1939.

■ Passing the National Board of Medical Examiners' exam within the previous 10 years allowed abridged licensure beginning in 1978.

■ Specialty Board Examinations and Certification began in 1936.

■ The Watson Clinic first required all physician partners to be specialty board-certified in January 1966. This was waived for two existing partners and, subsequently, for one partner of a medical group acquired in 1986.

■ In 1974, Watson Clinic physicians were required to meet the Florida Medical Association requirements for continuing medical education bi- or triennially. Clinic physicians subsequently came under state mandates, not only for hourly requirements but also for particular medical and sociological subject requirements to maintain state licensure.

Since the Clinic's inception, Clinic partners, in choosing new physicians, have evaluated their educational backgrounds, requiring educational documentation; licensure documentation; and personal and, in the past, credit references. Physician candidates are asked to submit three letters of recommendation that are verified with a personal phone call by a physician in the same department as the recruited physician. These letters become a permanent part of the personnel and credentialing file. The Watson Clinic has adopted LRMC's application procedures (figure 1, page 154). Candidates are chosen after extensive evaluation of educational and social background. The physician must be able to communicate effectively in English; proficiency in other languages is helpful. The clinic has learned from years of experience that the uniquely qualified individual will help create his or her own practice. The individual who does not measure up will detract from the hard-earned reputation of the group.

All candidates are evaluated over a 1-2 day period. It is not unusual to schedule two separate visits 6-8 weeks apart. The spouse is encouraged to be present so that he or she can observe and attempt to determine if living in the community will be enjoyable. The physician candidate is interviewed in a packed schedule, and emergencies or significant events are the only excuses available to participants. The candidate's and the interviewers' time is important, and the process is expensive to both the candidate and the Clinic.

The day may start with morning rounds at the hospital with a member of the prospective department. Afterward the prospective physician is transported to the clinic and undertakes 30-minute interviews with a cross-section of physician leaders and practitioners in a practice setting for the remainder of the day. He or she also meets and is expected to exchange information with

---

FIGURE 1. LAKELAND REGIONAL MEDICAL CENTER'S APPLICATION PROCESS

1. Medical school graduation.

2. Internship, residency, and fellowship programs; completion of an evaluation form is required.

3. All previous hospital and other health care facility affiliations; completion of an evaluation form is required.

4. Past malpractice history.

5. Malpractice insurance in the amount required by the hospital.

6. Current Florida medical license.

7. Current DEA registration.

8. Query from the American Medical Association.

9. Query received from the National Practitioner Data Bank.

10. Confirmation of board certification if applicable.

11. Other information that may be applicable for the specific physician.

12. Verification of any "gaps in time."

---

administrators, finance officers, and the Director of Risk Management. Conversations are open-ended, and frank queries are the cornerstone, as neither side needs subsequent surprises. A host physician escorts the candidate to lunch in the Library where he or she is able to converse with a number of physicians in a social setting. Dinners are in a comfortable conversational setting with 2-3 physicians and spouses.

Each interviewer submits a formal review of the candidate to the Medical Director, who has interviewed the candidate himself and summarizes the information. This process usually requires unanimous approval by the department, approval of the Executive Committee, and a partner vote by written or verbal response to that committee's minutes within five days. Ninety percent partner approval is required.

Spousal approval regarding the appointment is extremely important. The Clinic has lost a number of physicians later because of an unhappy spouse. Despite a fraternal and familial feeling within the group, and an attempt to provide a caring support system for the spouse, the Clinic family cannot cure homesickness. Loss of valuable caregivers affects a service, even when it is only temporary. This is an important profiling consideration.

With rare exceptions, physicians are accepted as employed associates for two years, after which time they are elected into full partnership. During this two-year period, the unified medical record as well as shared call schedules on both an inpatient and outpatient basis allow thorough evaluation of a physician by peers, section heads, the Medical Director, and the Clinic Chairman (CEO). In fact, all candidates are reviewed in the Partners Only Session of the bimonthly staff meeting. Approximately 75 percent of the associates complete the two years and become partners. Of the remaining 25 percent, approximately one-half elect to leave on their own because of dissatisfaction or undue expectations and the other half leave because partners and peers feel they should not be given a long-term commitment. There is only one level of partnership.

Credentialing and recredentialing of medical providers is maintained by the Contracting and Market Development Department. Watson Clinic also has a Credentialing Committee made up of six Watson Clinic physicians and administrative staff. This committee is responsible for recommendation of initial appointment, reappointment, or disciplinary action to the Board of Directors. Watson Clinic credentialing includes maintaining current and documented licensure, DEA registration, and malpractice insurance. At reappointment time, all dynamic information is reverified. Reappointment also includes member complaints, information specific to quality improvement and utilization management activities, medical records review, and site visit evaluations.

Profiling Clinic Physicians

The Watson Clinic Department of Quality Improvement established a plan for physician profiling in 1997. The plan was to select a variety of indicators of physician performance, to measure them on a regular basis, and to present a report to physicians on a monthly or quarterly basis. The types of data to be collected included:

■ Frequency and distribution of specialty specific diagnosis codes.

■ Frequency and distribution of specialty-specific performance codes.

■ Cost of laboratory services per major diagnosis code.

■ Cost of laboratory per major procedure code.

■ Patient satisfaction survey data.

■ Appointment availability.

■ Reception room delays.

■ Peer group analysis of compliance with practice guidelines.

In August 1997, the Watson Clinic Quality Improvement Department began analyzing data about frequency and cost of diagnoses and procedures by physicians. Counseling of physicians did bring about an improvement in appropriate coding and billing patterns. Watson Clinic has extensive analytical reports on its primary care physicians, the use of laboratory services, and referral services for two capitated contracts. At any time, Watson Clinic could extend that analysis to include all physicians and all patients, regardless of insurance contracts. The Watson Clinic Board of Directors has requested that the Board of Directors of LRMC consider supplying its unpublished quarterly CQI data on Clinic physicians.

Practice guidelines can improve the decision-making process. Many decisions physicians make are based on gut feelings, not on scientific facts. In 1997, in preparation for a managed care environment, Watson Clinic physicians began developing clinical guidelines on disease entities representing either high either high-volume or high-cost entities chosen by medical administration (figure 2, below). Physician teams in multiple specialties in conjunction with medical administration spent countless hours reviewing previously published protocols and regionalizing them to the Watson Clinic practice model. Approximately half of those guidelines were completed and approved by the appropriate departments. The other half is nearing completion. None have been implemented. The plan is to develop a compliance form for each practice guideline and to select a small number of charts for each physician covered by the practice guidelines. These charts will be reviewed by physicians in the same discipline to determine the degree of compliance with practice guidelines. Data would be collected and added to Clinic physician profiles.

Patient satisfaction is measurable. Until mid-1977, an oral patient satisfaction survey was conducted on each new physician prior to the vote for partnership. This information and the quarterly reports of patient complaints

FIGURE 2. PRIMARY CARE MANAGEMENT AND PRACTICE GUIDELINES

Bronchial Asthma	Depression	Orthopedic MRI	Peptic Ulcer
Allergic Rhinitis	Alzheimer's	Low Back Pain	Disease
Allergy Referral	Diabetes Mellitus	Pediatric	Athersclerotic
Breast Lump	Headaches	Bronchitis	Heart Disease
Childbirth	Hypertension	Pediatric Asthma	Congestive Heart
		Adult UTI	Failure
			Asymtomatic
			Patient

were reviewed as part of the physician's candidacy for partnership. The Clinic has actively carried out patient satisfaction surveys on other physicians for more than 10 years. This information is disseminated to the department, the Board, and the individual physician. In 1997, we began performing patient satisfaction surveys on patients cared for by all Watson Clinic physicians in every Watson Clinic location. In addition to surveys, we collect reports on patients' complaints and requests for changes of physician. Also data were collected on availability of appointments for each physician and on typical reception room waiting times.

Patient complaints are monitored on a monthly basis. All physicians' personal information regarding numbers and types of complaints and how they are handled are circulated quarterly to physicians. In addition, an annual summary is sent in a coded manner so that a physician may compare him- or herself to peers regarding number and types of administrative complaints that have been received. Profiling is conducted to assess health care, physician compliance, and good citizenship and as an economic credentialing tool.

Beginning in 1990, patients requesting a change of physician in a department were required to fill out a Change of Physician form. Initially, both physicians had to sign off on this request, but, since 1996, physicians are no longer a part of the administrative process. Each physician's activity-attitude, fee, delay/wait, policy, care, notify, excess tests, service, access, billing, and other-is kept in the database, which is reviewed by the CQI and Executive committees. The Clinic monitors the number of patients who have changed physicians and periodically circulates this information to physicians. Physicians who are outliers are counseled.

In 1997, a "Physician Report Card" was developed. The criteria are still in the fledgling stages but include charges, RVUs, and visits per day; paid support staff hours per visit; and relative value units per visit. The Clinic is attempting to add physician colleague satisfaction, patient satisfaction, and resource utilization criteria to the report card. These changes are driven by Watson Clinic desire for high-quality medical care; patient satisfaction; and, ultimately, clinic profitability.

Collection, interpretation, and dissemination of all such collected data are the responsibility of the Director of Quality Improvement and Risk Management, who reports to the Medical Director and the Clinical Leadership Council, the latter made up of spokespersons of every department. Both the Council, which is chaired by the Medical Director, and the Medical Director report to the Board of Directors.

Watson Clinic continues to monitor sources of revenue by physicians on a monthly basis. After application of various taxing procedures depending on materials, space, and personnel costs, a physician production credit is established. This figure is used to enter data into a complex formula based on equality, longevity, and productivity, ultimately determining physician incomes.

Hospital Physician Profiling

For many years, the only requirement for practice at LRMC was a certificate of graduation from an accredited medical school and a license granted by the Florida Board of Medical Examiners. However, to obtain that license, a physician had to successfully complete a State of Florida Basic Science Examination and pass the Florida Board of Medical Examiners examination. Beginning in 1978, passing one of the examinations of the National Board of Medical Examiners sufficed. Foreign medical graduates were required to pass the Educational Commission for Foreign Medical Graduates (ECFMG) examination beginning in the 1970s.

Hospital credentialing at LRMC begins with a preapplication that is used to obtain preliminary information on potential applicants. LRMC's formal application procedure then requires extensive documentation (figure 1, page 154) that must be verified directly from the source. This requires a significant commitment of time and effort by administration and the medical staff.

Results of this process are reviewed formally by an LRMC Credentials Committee, the Medical Executive Committee, and the Board of Directors. The medical staff bylaws require board certification in order to be appointed to the medical staff except in the case of recent graduates of training programs, in which case the physician has five years to obtain board certification. The physician's total credentialing file must demonstrate that he or she is "above average." Once a physician is appointed to the medical staff, there is the usual monitoring of practices through the quality improvement process and by the Risk Management Department.

LRMC compiles a quarterly report of physician CQI activity. The report includes surgical morbidity and mortality, physician medical procedure morbidity and mortality, and other morbidity and mortality data available concerning the medical staff, including Watson Clinic physicians.

While hospitals were increasing their use of CQI, some hospitals also began to discuss economic profiling of physicians as a way to improve their economic vitality. That was never an issue at LRMC. Although LRMC does not economically privilege physicians, economic data are provided to physicians for comparison purposes.

Starting in 1986, regional Watson Clinic physicians have also practiced at hospitals in Bartow, Lake Wales, Plant City, and Brandon, Florida. These hospitals monitor their physicians and medical and surgical care with tools similar to those used by LRMC.

Into the Future-Our New Tools

Clearly, there is a "big brother" element to physician profiling that makes some physicians uncomfortable. Watson Clinic physicians recognize that we must profile ourselves accurately. We are already being profiled by major insurance groups; local, state, and federal governments; and a number of watchdog groups. We must not be at the mercy of outside entities by accepting their potentially biased and inaccurate performance information. The physicians of the Watson Clinic believe that it is in our strategic interest to collect valid information and be able to share it with potential purchasers of our services.

New tools to improve physician profiling will be necessary. There must be new methods of collecting data, including difficult direct observation. Because of the volume of data involved in physician profiling, automation is essential. Our computer systems have become increasingly powerful, efficient, and sophisticated. They allow collection, collation, storage, interpretation, and dissemination of pertinent data. An IDX practice management software system installed in the Clinic in November 1998 will lead to enhancement of data collection and availability.

Watson Clinic has purchased an electronic medical record from Shared Medical Systems (SMS). When fully functional, it will be able to measure compliance with practice guidelines automatically and consistently. The Clinic has purchased new appointment scheduling software that is designed to automatically collect data about appointment availability and reception room delays. It has also purchased new billing software from IDX that will allow us to analyze the financial performance of each physician for each diagnosis and procedure code. Profiling capabilities to measure a physician's necessary compliance with practice guidelines is probably to be expected.

The Watson Clinic will continue to refine and update its profiling mechanisms. In spite of extensive application and evaluation forms, surveys, and computer databases, Watson Clinic physicians, working together and evaluating candidates and one another one-on-one, will probably continue to be the Clinic's best profiling tool.

References

1. Annis, J. *History of the Watson Clinic.* Lakeland, Fla.: Watson Clinic, 1981, pp. 1-2.

2. Uzych, L. "The Promise and Challenge of Physician Profiling." *Nebraska Medical Journal* 79(8):298-9, Aug. 1994.

Angelo P. Spoto Jr., MD, FACP, is a Partner, Watson Clinic LLP, Lakeland, Florida. He is Past President of the Watson Clinic Foundation and of the American Medical Group Association.

Acknowledgment: The following talented colleagues graciously shared with me their experience, written thoughts, and ideas. At the Watson Clinic, Dale Taylor, MD; Stephen Flax, MD; Robert H. Chapman, MD, PhD.; Glen Garden, MD; Jorge Gonzalez, MD; Paul Bresnan, MD; Fran Hamm, RN; Mary Ann Blanchard, RN; Mary Wicker, RN; Elaine Bertles, MPH; Stephanie Guice, BA; Sharon Paul, BA; Julie Roberson, BS, MS; Cheryl Dee, PhD; and Chad Waldron, BA; and, at LRMC, Edwin Sammer, MD; Elena Mesa, CMSC; and Jack Stephens, MHA.

CHAPTER 10

Physician Profiling in Managed Care Organizations
by John M. Ludden, MD, CPE, FACPE

A physician profiling system is a detailed reflection of the purpose of a managed health care system. The purpose is, in turn, conditioned by the history of the organization that the managed system serves. This brief report is intended to describe the development of physician profiling at one managed care organization and to highlight some general issues for physician executives in their potential involvement in similar efforts.

Harvard Pilgrim Health Care (HPHC) was formed in 1993 through the merger of Harvard Community Health Plan (HCHP), a staff and group network model HMO, and Pilgrim Health Care (PHC), an IPA model. The long-range mission of the organization is improvement of the health of society. HCHP brought to the merger a history of group practice-based clinical quality improvement. PHC brought a strong network culture critically attuned to the use of data and information formulated on a practice-by-practice basis.

With a strong group practice culture and an exclusive delivery system-insurance company relationship, HCHP had moved away from individual practice profiles toward a system of goals, targets, and measurements based on practice group responsibility for productivity, quality, and outcomes. Incentive and physician evaluation systems were keyed to the achievement of performance targets at the aggregate level. For example, achievement of budget and quality targets (e.g., immunization rates) were assessed at a department and then a health center level, using the automated medical record as a core clinical information system.

The individual practice culture of PHC made reporting of individual practice performance a critical delivery system feature and a major tool for medical management of the system. As in most network model plans, Pilgrim physicians have multiple HMO relationships. In Massachusetts, these are discounted fee-for-service arrangements that employ withholds and other appended risk-sharing arrangements and that are managed through a claims-based information system. Development of practice-specific information was a very important feature of the PHC delivery system.

After the merger and in the context of important information system issues, HPHC temporarily suspended the sending out of practice profiles that PHC had been accustomed to receiving. The issues of system compatibility, functionality, and capacity proved central in the decision. The network side of the delivery organization began to push for more such utilization information and for the information to be gathered and structured for ease of use.

As part of an ongoing effort to understand and reduce medical costs while improving quality, a specific business plan was developed to search for opportunities for cost reduction through improved clinical management of ambulatory care, inpatient care, and pharmaceuticals. With a strong tradition in clinical quality improvement, HCHP brought to the table sophistication in the array and use of clinical information that could be focused on clinical conditions of high population prevalence, such as heart disease and diabetes. For both group-model delivery systems and the network, the program was designed to allow analysis of practice patterns in terms of utilization and expenditures. The role of the physician profile is to provide the delivery system with tools to help manage the clinical practice through peer comparison at a group and individual level. The uses of such information will necessarily differ, depending on whether the delivery system sees itself as a group practice or whether the focus of attention is on individual physicians.

HPHC decided that the physician profiling system should be rebuilt after the merger so that it expanded in scope and served both medical management and utilization monitoring functions more effectively. While it might have been possible to develop the profiling system internally, it seemed more expedient to search for an outside vendor, especially considering the continued systems issues. In a first step, purchasing specifications were developed in close collaboration with the network delivery system and included the following important areas:

■ Data integration capacity.

■ Case-mix adjustment.

■ Ability to review individual cases over a continuum of time and location.

■ Software applications allowing generation of useful reports.

After evaluation, Practice Patterns Science* was chosen to develop the system for HPHC's use.

An important feature of the preparation for use of the new profiling system was examination and development of supporting internal policies. Without internal policies and procedures, profiling data would have no guidance or direction. At HPHC, a major corporate goal was to develop well-aligned relationships with physicians and other providers. The intent is not to use profiling to exercise health plan watchdog functions. Therefore, information on a particular physician's utilization experience is not the focus of the health plan at a corporate level. Rather, this information is fed back through the local practice leader. An elaborate policy system was designed to allay concerns (especially prominent in the group practices) about the use of practice-specific data for judgments about particular physicians. At the same time, it was well recognized that data and information would be used at the first level of medical management as a tool to improve practice quality and to decrease unnecessary expense.

At the aggregate level, practice patterns are identified and can be analyzed for intervention. The chief criteria for intervention include the importance of the practice pattern either financially or clinically and the amount of variation that is present in the whole collection of practices. Such interventions include establishing simple awareness of deviation from statistical norms of practice; focused education (such as "academic detailing" by established clinical leaders); broader educational efforts designed around clinical guidelines and pathways; and systematic practice changes that could be instituted for a group. For example, unusually high utilization of skull x-rays in sinusitis might result in any of these four interventions. Because excess utilization will be linked to improved financial performance in most of the reimbursement models used by HPHC, the financial incentive will be present, although it will not always be a primary issue. Some interventions may, in fact, add costs in the short range.

This general direction may not fit other managed care organizations or delivery systems. It is possible to develop profiling systems whose intent includes economic profiling, short-term cost reduction, etc. These systems were not included in the HPHC approach, even though it is the conviction of physician executives that reduction in variation in practice pattern will improve costs and quality of care overall and over time.

---

*The physician profiling system and the various related reports described in this chapter are proprietary to Practice Patterns, Inc., St. Louis, Missouri, and may not be used without its permission.

The profiling system is a specialty-based report that includes the top 24-28 conditions that account for 70-80 percent of primary care "episodes of care." These conditions are determined pragmatically. High-volume conditions, such as sinusitis, hypertension, and upper respiratory infections, are assessed for their comparative resource consumption by an individual practice. For an individual provider or a practice leader, this approach results in an ability to compare a practitioner's frequency for a given intervention (e.g., skull x-ray for sinusitis) with that of peers and to the assess the financial impact of any variation. The information system allows identification of statistical under-utilization as well as utilization in excess of the peer experience.

While measurement of utilization and the design of interventions are critical, HPHC has also found that timely reporting of data and adequate attention to the design of the "display" of information are also of central importance. Continuous improvement of the information display is important, and it is highly unlikely that a delivery system will get this right the first time. Physicians and their practices are major stakeholders in the use of data and will require more than a single "data dump" from the insurer.

Each communication with a physician emphasizes that (in HPHC's case) the information is intended to be educational and confidential (with explicit limits if appropriate). Further, the cover letter describes the scope of the data used for the report, the sources of data, the sources of systematic error, and the intent of the program, which is to "...identify medical conditions for which your use of resources appears to be substantially different from your peers'." At the end of each physician report, a series of "Questions and Answers" cover questions about the origin, purpose; access, accuracy, meaning, and uses of the report. Also included are intervention resources available to the physician from HPHC.

The report itself is a graphic and tabular display of several "cuts" of the indi-vidual physician's data. First, a four-quadrant display describes "Resource Allocation by Medical Condition." This is followed by "Resource Allocation by Service Category" and a table of "Statistically Significant Procedure Variations" for both ambulatory and inpatient portions of care.

The data and information are displayed for each physician and for aggregates of the delivery system. A simplified example for a physician is shown in figure 1, page 165. In the full display, all of the most common conditions are shown (if the physician treats enough cases for each condition). The figure is accom-panied by an extensive description of its construction. The array allows a physician to see where his or her practice and patient population may vary from peer averages. The general area around the center is not much different from peer practice. One area of importance to the organization will be the

FIGURE 1. RESOURCE ALLOCATION BY MEDICAL CONDITION

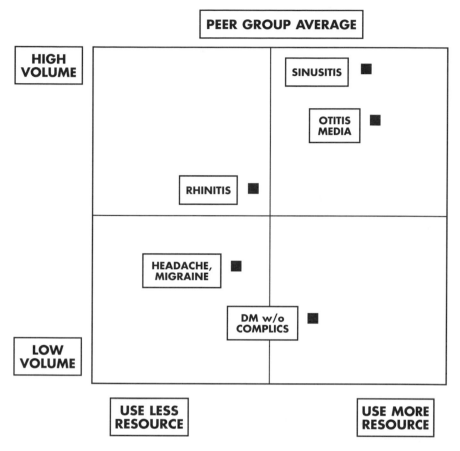

high-volume/more-resource quadrant. This graphic encourages a physician to drill down into the data but still presents enough of a "big picture" to give perspective and to remain nonjudgmental.

A second graphic describes "Resource Allocation by Service Category" for an individual physician compared to the peer group average (figure 2, page 166). For physicians more inclined to think in categorical terms, this may prove a useful characterization of practice. The gray bar describes the total range of experience, while the white internal bar represents the middle 70th percentile in utilization performance. The black oval denotes the individual physician's results.

Finally, a table describes "Statistically Significant Procedure Variations," together with their cost impact. The sample table on page 166 describes a few areas in which the profiled physician is at some variation from the peer group average and points to the potential for studying the practice further, with the understanding that "statistical significance is not the same as clinical meaning.

FIGURE 2. RESOURCE ALLOCATION BY SERVICE CATEGORY

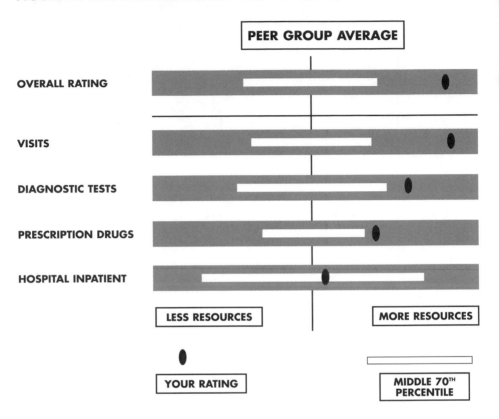

AMBULATORY-OUTPATIENT VISITS

Medical Condition	Procedure Group	# of Services	Services Per Episode			
			You	Peers	Percentage	Impact
Sinusitis	Tympanometry	54	1.644	0.183	>500%	$1,300
Sinusitis	Skull x-ray	82	0.271	0.005	>500%	$3,600
Otitis Media	Skull x-ray	10	0.108	0.002	>500%	$ 450

The full report tabulates data in each of the areas of resource use: outpatient visits, outpatient laboratory, outpatient diagnostic tests, outpatient medical and surgical procedures, outpatient prescription drugs, inpatient services, outpatient facilities, inpatient facilities, alternative sites, and "other." This enables focus on areas in which resource use is less or greater than the peer group average.

As with any systematic intervention in medical management, cost and return are important to assess as completely as possible. The costs of developing and implementing a profiling system go beyond simple information system expense and include initial policy definition, collaboration required for implementation, design of the information and data display vehicles, and appropriate training of the users. Beyond those initial expenses, interventions, physician outreach, and education required to change practice patterns all require additional resources.

To be effective, a profiling system needs to have an appropriate return on investment (ROI). At its stage of implementation in 1998, the HPHC profiling system had not yet achieved a positive ROI. We know that some of the return will be very hard to quantity in our delivery models, although we expect to be able to document aggregate changes in practice patterns and to infer savings and quality improvements. Some of the yield from a profiling system will be increased utilization of certain interventions (e.g., mammography), and result in immediate cost increases whose ultimate financial payback may accrue at another place and in another time. It is important to be clear on what payback is expected, when it will accrue, and whether it will be directly quantifiable.

In conclusion, the HPHC experience with physician profiling suggests that there are several important development criteria for a managed care organization to consider:

■ The purpose of the profiling system should be tied to the purpose of the organization.

■ The system should be carefully specified, in collaboration with practicing physicians and clinical leaders wherever possible.

■ The uses of data should be governed by clear policies and procedures.

■ The menu of interventions should be understood by the organization and its associated physicians.

■ Adequate attention must be paid to design, display, and distribution of timely data.

■ ROI should be explicitly analyzed, with special attention to including all of the resources that may be required to produce practice changes.

John M. Ludden, MD, CPE, FACPE, was Senior vice President for Medical Affairs, Harvard Pilgrim Health Care, at the time this chapter was written. He is now Associate Clinical Professor, Department of Ambulatory Care and Preventive Medicine, Harvard Medical School, Boston, Massachusetts.

CHAPTER 11

Profiling at the Department of Veterans Affairs
by James Tuchschmidt, MD, MBA, and
Carol M. Ashton, MD, MPH

*F*our years ago, the Department of Veterans Affairs (VA) embarked on the awesome process of redefining and reengineering health care for veterans. The blueprint for the new VA attempts to ensure a seamless continuum of care that balances health maintenance, disease prevention, and a population perspective with the episodic treatment of acute disease. Eligibility reform legislation indemnified care for eligible veterans who enroll with the VA, offering access to a comprehensive and uniform set of health care benefits. Our system has been redesigned to be more patient-centered and customer-focused. New organizational structures and performance systems promote responsibility and accountability for managing scarce resources as well as health care outcomes.

Medical center performance data published during the first few years of this reorganization had a profound impact on overall system performance.[1] It was clear, however, that these performance expectations had to be more compelling at the provider level. Numerous grassroots efforts began to take shape within VA's 22 integrated networks, and a decision was made to unify them into one national model. Much of our approach nationally to practice profiling is based on what was learned from pilot projects in these pioneering networks, particularly the Northwest Network (VISN20). In this chapter, we detail our approach to practice profiling and articulate our future practice management strategies. At the risk of being redundant, we would like to begin by exploring several important principles VA considered when crafting a practice profiling system.

Practice Management Principals Adopted by VA
In 1982, Wennberg and Gittelsohn reported significant variation in the utilization of surgical procedures by physicians in the northeastern United

States—variability that could not be explained by demographic differences.[2] Since then, numerous other investigators have found significant small area variation in the utilization of health care resources, and presumably the cost of care, with no demonstrable corresponding variation in outcome quality. Indeed, researchers have at best been able to explain only about 35 percent of this variation on the basis of disease burden. Many other factors besides severity of illness may contribute to the variation seen in clinical utilization, including socioeconomic characteristics that influence care-seeking behavior, availability of services in the community, out-of-pocket costs born by the patient, chance variation, and certainly the practice patterns of physicians.

Numerous efforts have been employed to alter physician practice patterns—continuing medical education, use of opinion leaders, mentoring, performance feedback, prompts and reminders, and incentives and sanctions. Most of these measures, when used in isolation, have failed to alter practice patterns or have achieved only modest (10-15 percent) benefits. However, some important conclusions can be drawn from this literature. First, multi-faceted approaches are likely to produce sustainable change. Greco and Eisenberg showed that using a combination of methods to influence physician behavior (education, feedback, physician participation, administrative rules and reminders, and financial incentives) is more effective than using any single approach.[3] Second, real-time intervention at the point of decision making probably has the greatest impact. Furthermore, Tompkins et al. believe that, "In medical groups, profiling can help individual members to become more committed to group norms....Groups achieve a sense of community by leading individual practitioners to identify with common goals and practice norms."[4]

VA developed its practice management strategies with these principles in mind. Currently, we only provide periodic feedback to clinicians, and data are intended only for quality improvement purposes. We have developed acceptable case-mix adjustment methodologies, which we will discuss here in more detail. As our information systems mature, we plan to link performance data with real-time prompts and alerts. We may ultimately institute some form of performance-based remuneration, once we are satisfied with the quality of our data. To guide these efforts, we developed a list of critical attributes we thought desirable in any profiling product (table 1, page 171).

If they are to accept profiles, providers must believe that the parameters being profiled are both reliable and valid. Reliability refers to the accuracy and completeness of the data and to their reproducibility over time. Validity, on the other hand, reflects the degree to which a parameter measures what is intended. If the profiles are used for decision making or are linked to compensation, they should withstand a higher degree of analytic scrutiny than if

---

TABLE 1. CRITICAL ATTRIBUTES FOR PRACTICE PROFILING

- Data integrity, reliability, and validity
- Standardized data sets
- Timeliness of feedback
- Longitudinal data
- Decomposable data sets
- Cost and quality outcomes
- Case-mix adjustment
- Sphere of influence
- Clear line of sight
- Anonymity and confidentiality

---

they are used only for screening purposes. Missing or inaccurate data elements, particularly from claims-based sources, can be very problematic. Noteworthy in this respect is Iezzoni's research demonstrating how the failure to accurately code comorbidities can lead to improbable risk assessments of inpatient mortality rates.[5] Furthermore, we recognized the need to standardize data elements and definitions across the country so that we could aggregate data at various levels of the organization in order to compare geographic regions and to establish benchmarks.

The third attribute, timeliness, has two dimensions for our purposes. First, we believe that profiles should reflect current practice and attempt to minimize the lag between data collection and reporting. Second, the feedback itself should be timely. Feedback that is timely and clinically meaningful will increase the significance of the information. Thus, feedback provided at the point of decision making, particularly when combined with prompts, will probably be most effective at changing practice patterns. For example, we are developing computerized clinical alerts that will notify the primary care provider that the patient is in need of a routine mammogram and, at the same time, provide feedback on the rate at which screening mammography is performed for his or her panel of patients.

Furthermore, the methodology should account, we believe, for variations in severity of illness, particularly when relatively small populations are being compared. Indeed, every effort should be made to control or explain as much of the variation between providers as possible. One of the most significant sources of variation in our system, particularly with respect to productivity measures, is the amount of time dedicated to the activity being profiled. For example, many of our primary care clinicians also have specialty practices or are engaged in academic activities. Therefore, any profiling system we developed had to account for the time allocated to activities of interest in order to represent a clinician's entire contribution fairly.

Furthermore, small provider panels will inherently have greater chance variation in most normative-based parameters than will larger sized panels. Consequently, panel size had to be considered in any statistical analysis.

The next three attributes refer to database architecture, and two of them-longitudinal analysis and decomposable data sets-enhance profiling as a quality management tool. The inclusion of longitudinal data allows providers to visualize changes in practice effectiveness over time, while decomposable data sets allow outliers to investigate root causes. Furthermore, we wanted to ensure that data were presented in a way that maintained provider confidentiality and that our database employed acceptable mechanisms to allow access only to authorized individuals.

Finally, profiles are developed to produce actionable feedback. The last two attributes relate to the ability of providers to alter performance outcomes. We felt strongly that providers must be able to influence the process of care being measured (Sphere of Influence) and clearly understand how their behavior affects the desired outcome (Clear Line of Sight). This is not to imply that clinicians need to entirely control the process of care, but rather that the provider must be able to influence the outcome in some meaningful way. Furthermore, while performance data can be developed at the team or the group practice level, aggregate feedback is meaningful only if the individuals within the group can relate their performance to that of the group as a whole or to a clear norm or standard. Feedback lacking these characteristics is likely to lead only to frustration and disregard for the entire performance measurement system.[6]

Intended Purposes

Practice profiling is an analytic tool that uses epidemiological methods to compare providers on various dimensions by focusing on patterns of care for defined populations of patients over time rather than on individual occurrences of care.[7] VA has instituted practice profiling as part of its practice management strategy in order to:

■ Link individual performance to corporate goals aimed at improving the five domains of health care value (technical quality, patient satisfaction, functional outcomes, access, and cost).

■ Enable leaders to clarify expectations and performance accountability at the provider and team levels.

■ Enable providers and teams to learn about their practices and discover opportunities for improvement.

■ Facilitate a learning- and performance-oriented culture.

Fundamentally, we view practice profiling as a valuable quality improvement tool. By assessing morbidity, mortality, and other outcome proxies, VA hopes to improve quality, reduce utilization of inappropriate care, and increase utilization of underutilized services. Future refinements of our practice management systems will attempt to link resource utilization to outcomes for specific conditions that are relevant to a particular patient population. We also hope to be able to focus numerous management activities in more cost-effective ways. For example, utilization review systems have traditionally employed onerous preauthorization and concurrent review processes indiscriminately. Practice profiling has allowed us to focus utilization review efforts in a more efficient and a less intrusive manner by concentrating these activities on clinicians whose practice patterns deviate from stated goals or norms. Furthermore, traditional utilization management has concentrated on identifying outliers, whereas our profiling efforts attempt to change practice norms.

At this time, we have limited formal use of the data to quality improvement activities and have imposed specific prohibitions against using the data explicitly for performance assessment or remuneration. We believe that practice management data will be inherently suspect during the early stages of this initiative. Data integrity, data validity, measure definitions, and analytic techniques are not likely to be refined enough that our practice management reports can be used for these purposes. At some point, however, we may link practice profile data to incentives. Critics of cost-driven profiles identify a very real danger of incentives to underserve patients. Indeed, VA faces significant challenges in rationalizing unnecessarily complex and costly services in an effort to provide a greater breadth of care to more veterans. In addition to restricting use of these data, we have attempted to balance cost and quality measures in an effort to

---

TABLE 2. MEASURES INCLUDED ON PRACTICE MANAGEMENT REPORTS

- Primary care panel size
- BDOC/1000 unique patients/year
- Encounters/unique patient/year
- Prescription costs/unique patient/month
- Lab costs/unique patient/month
- Imaging costs/unique patient/month
- % unique patients over age 65 yrs who have received influenza vaccination
- % unique patients over age 65 yrs who have received pneumococcal vaccination
- % of unique patients with diabetes who have HbA1C's measured within last year
- % of unique patients with ischemic heart disease who are on ASA
- % of unique patients with coronary artery atherosclerosis who have LDL < 130
- % of unique patients with a history of congestive heart failure who are on an ACE inhibitor

mitigate these concerns. When compensation is tied to performance, Shapiro and colleagues argue, incentives should be based on the performance of small groups of providers or teams. "Incentives targeted to an individual physician affect individual patient care decisions more strongly than incentives conditioned on group performance. However, the latter is less strongly tied to the care of any individual patient than the former and may stimulate collective action to reduce costs."[8]

Practice Management Reports

As a general rule, the parameters profiled measure cost, service, quality, or productivity and reflect the process, the organization, or the outcome of care. The measures currently profiled or under consideration are listed in table 2, page 173. We have chosen to profile rate-based comparative information reflecting either normative practice patterns or standards-based measures. We recognize that practice-based norms may not necessarily reflect appropriate care (see figure 1, below). For example, preventive health services, such as colon cancer screening, may be rendered at a uniformly low rate. Consequently, a comparison of individual practitioner against mean group performance may be misleading. Therefore, we have attempted to link numerous parameters to practice guidelines in an effort to develop standards-based measures. Furthermore, guidelines help practitioners distinguish appropriate from inappropriate approaches to care. Without such guidance, performance measurement systems are likely to alter both inappropriate and appropriate uses of services, particularly when linked to financial incentives.[8]

We electronically distribute reports containing observed and expected data for each measure, along with a statistical assessment of outlier status. Expected data for normative measures is calculated using regression techniques to adjust for differences in illness burden among patients. These models usually have adjusted r^2 between 0.3 and 0.4. Drill down and analytic capability is available using standard on-line analytical processing software (figures 2-5, pages 175-178). Through this Web-like interface, managers and clinicians can explore the detailed information underlying most measures. For example, one can drill down into observed and expected pharmacy cost data to compare groups by

---

FIGURE 1. PRACTICE PROFILING
Data and Measures

⊃ Normative or Practice-based Parameters
⊃ Standards-Based Parameters

✓ Practice-based parameters may not always reflect appropriate care. For example, clinicians may render preventive health services at a uniformly low rate!

FIGURE 2

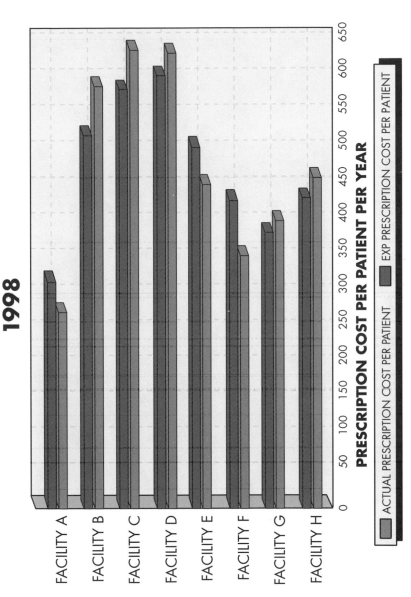

PRESCRIPTION COST PER PATIENT BY FACILITY 1998

FIGURE 3

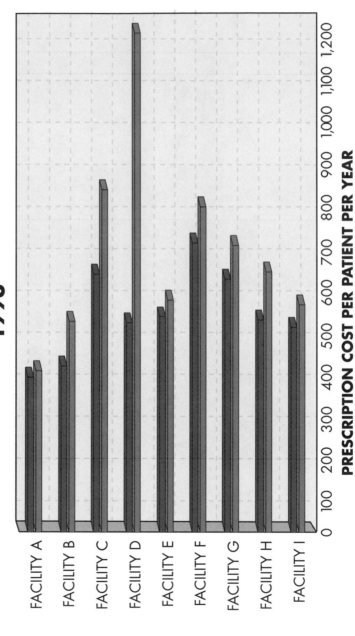

PRESCRIPTION COST PER PATIENT BY PROVIDER 1998

FIGURE 4

1998 PRESCRIPTION COSTS FOR PROVIDER 75865

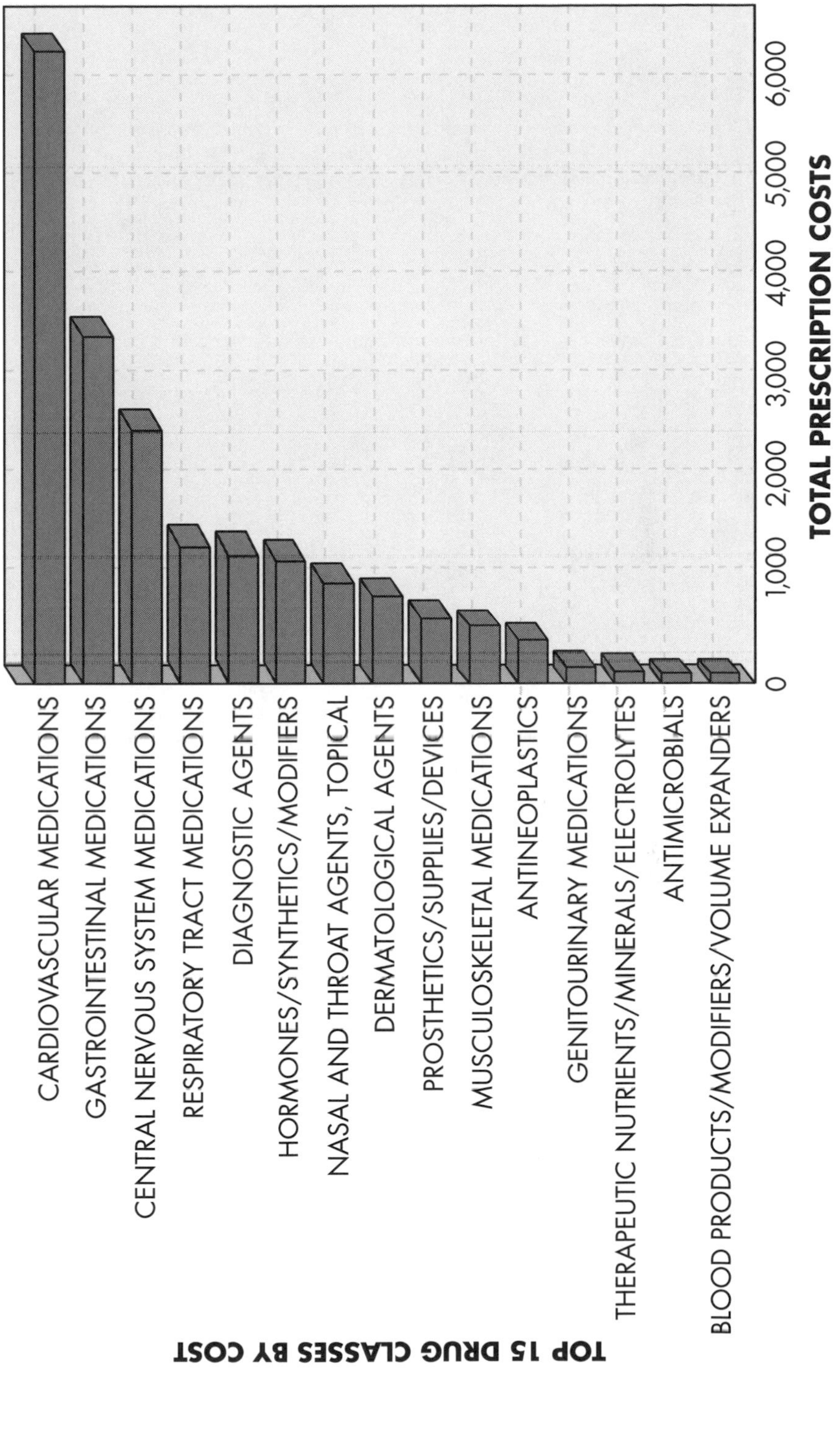

TOP 15 DRUG CLASSES BY COST

CARDIOVASCULAR MEDICATIONS

GASTROINTESTINAL MEDICATIONS

CENTRAL NERVOUS SYSTEM MEDICATIONS

RESPIRATORY TRACT MEDICATIONS

DIAGNOSTIC AGENTS

HORMONES/SYNTHETICS/MODIFIERS

NASAL AND THROAT AGENTS, TOPICAL

DERMATOLOGICAL AGENTS

PROSTHETICS/SUPPLIES/DEVICES

MUSCULOSKELETAL MEDICATIONS

ANTINEOPLASTICS

GENITOURINARY MEDICATIONS

THERAPEUTIC NUTRIENTS/MINERALS/ELECTROLYTES

ANTIMICROBIALS

BLOOD PRODUCTS/MODIFIERS/VOLUME EXPANDERS

TOTAL PRESCRIPTION COSTS

0   1,000   2,000   3,000   4,000   5,000   6,000

FIGURE 5

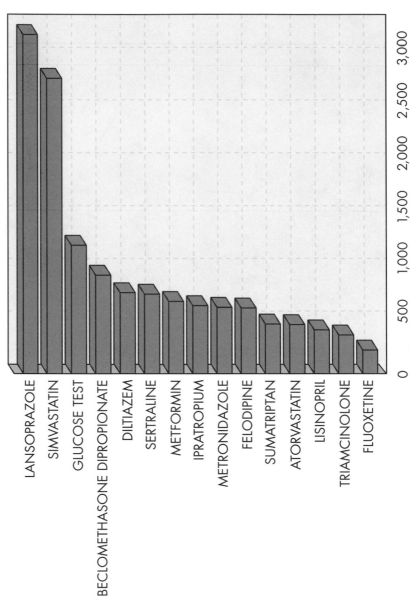

TOP 15 DRUGS BY 1998 COST FOR PROVIDER 75865

facility or individual practitioners or subsets of patients. With this point and click interface, one can then determine the classes of drugs being prescribed that contribute to the overall prescription costs of a provider panel.

Case Mix Adjustment

We have developed and validated a risk-adjustment model for our veteran population that minimizes the influence of known factors on our peer-to-peer comparisons. From the outset, we considered this an extremely important part of our strategy. The models we have developed allow us to publish valid expected outcomes, which clinicians can use to compare their actual performance to that of their peers. Risk adjustment is a process in which epidemiological and statistical techniques are used to standardize extraneous factors across populations or samples of patients so that between-group differences in outcome rates, including rates of health services use, can be attributed more validly to a hypothesized cause—in this case, practice style. Risk adjustment can be used to remove or minimize variation introduced by known factors and may be particularly critical when the populations compared are very small or very heterogeneous. The variation remaining after risk adjustment may be due solely to differences in the process of care, but it may also be due to unknown patient or population characteristics.

Thus, two broad categories of factors predominantly drive complication rates or utilization outcomes-patient-related factors that are not under the control of the medical provider or health care system (for example, age and diagnosis) and process-of-care factors that can often be modified.[9] With respect to practice profiling, we hypothesize that between-practice differences in outcome rates are attributable to practice style or local system inefficiencies. The unchangeable patient-related factors, although they have significant influence on outcome rates, are extraneous and therefore are the focus of risk adjustment. Each patient, and by extension each practice, has a particular configuration of unchangeable patient-related factors that constitute a risk for a certain outcome. By controlling for differences in illness burden across clinically dissimilar groups of patients, risk-adjustment procedures allow the influence of medical practice (quality, efficiency, etc.) to become more apparent. The between-practice variability that remains after risk adjustment may be attributed to factors under the practitioner's control.

Statistical methods of risk adjustment are unnecessary when certain kinds of rates are tracked within categories of patients. For example, there is no need to use statistical techniques to adjust for between-practice rates of influenza vaccination in people over age 65. Creating the cohort or the category is risk adjustment enough, because there is agreement that the target rate for this standards-based measure is 100 percent. However, many outcome measures do not fit so neatly into such categories, nor can there be agreement about the right target rate. For example, what is the "right" hospitalization rate in people over age 65 with community-acquired pneumonia? The "right" length of stay? The "right" case fatality rate?

Thus, in comparing outcomes across non-randomly assigned groups of patients, risk adjustment is necessary whenever patient-related factors strongly influence a rate and whenever the "right" rate cannot be known. When rates are compared across relatively small groups, as in practice profiling, risk adjustment becomes even more critical. Small sample sizes almost always mean greater heterogeneity with regard to measurable demographic and clinical features and with regard to unmeasured patient factors that drive rates (e.g., compliance). Decades of experience and research have shown that intensity of hospital use increases with age and differs by diagnosis (as does the risk of death). The differences in service use and one-year survival rates between patients with osteoarthritis and patients with small cell lung cancer are a case in point. Different types of patients gravitate to different types of clinicians, even within the same specialty. A comparison of crude (unadjusted) hospital use rates or death rates between practices gives no useful information about the quality or the efficiency of medical care in those practices and may be misleading. Indeed, demographic and diagnostic factors are far more powerful influences on patients' use of health services and their probability of dying in a certain time interval.

Many approaches have been developed to account for demographic and diagnostic differences among patients in the ambulatory setting.[10] These patient classifications are based in part on past resource consumption, such as the Ambulatory Patient Groups,[11] or on disease burden, such as the Ambulatory Care Groups (ACG) developed by Jonathan Weiner and others at Johns Hopkins University.[12] The ACG system classifies patients on the basis of age, gender, type of diagnosis, and number of diagnoses into mutually exclusive and exhaustive groups, the members of which are expected to have similar health services use. In selecting an approach, we decided against using a system based on resource consumption for two reasons. First, these methods seem to be based on circular reasoning ("my patients must be sicker because I use more resources," which may or may not be true). Second, because resource use is a function of unchangeable patient factors as well as practice style, any risk adjustment based on resource use has the unfortunate effect of statistically removing the effects of the very factor of most interest: practice style.

Patient classification systems simply put patients into groups; risk adjustment requires that those groups be used in statistical models. We use ACGs as indicator variables in multivariable models. The particular model chosen depends on the nature of the utilization outcome variable that is under consideration. For example, in risk-adjusting hospital bed-day rates across panels, we use a two-stage model.[13] The first-stage model estimates the proportions of patients who have any hospital use at all (less than 20 percent do), and the second-stage model estimates the levels of bed-day rates for those who did use a hospital during the period. Choosing the appropriate statistical model, calibrating it appropriately, and then assessing its fit are matters for statisticians or epidemiologists. However, most aspects of statistical modeling for risk adjustment of practice profiles are well developed and within the expertise of nearly all methodologists.

The claim is often leveled that risk adjustment of practice profiles should be avoided or cannot be done, because the science of risk adjustment is not up to the task. This is the same as saying that practice profiles based on crude rates tell us what we need to know, namely, the extent to which practices are falling within some norm. We disagree! Given the overwhelming, consistent evidence that health services use and outcomes vary more because of patient demographics and clinical attributes than as a result of the medical care system and individual practice style, we think between-practice utilization or outcome rates are at best uninterpretable and at worst misleading if they are not risk-adjusted. For example, we evaluated utilization of mental health inpatient bed days of care per thousand patients for a number of VA medical centers. The rank order of facilities was significantly different when based on risk-adjusted utilization versus unadjusted data. It is true that some aspects of multivariable statistical modeling are highly technical and difficult to understand without statistical training. However, the science is well developed. Risk adjustment has been around for more than 50 years, beginning with epidemiological comparisons of age- or sex-adjusted death rates across different groups of people.

The other argument that is raised is that risk adjustment does not or cannot work because available data sources do not capture all relevant risk variables. It is true that sources of data for risk adjustment-clinical charts or claims data-do not capture information on all the influences on service use or outcome (e.g., compliance, health beliefs, or genetic predisposition to disease). Data sources are improving all the time, however, and this will provide opportunities for researchers to study which of these factors carry the most weight. Even so, it is likely that age, gender, diagnosis, and total disease burden—variables available in many of today's clinical data systems, including those of the VA—will be found important. Risk adjustment of certain utilization and outcome rates is essential for valid comparisons across practices.

Lessons Learned

We continue to face numerous obstacles in implementing practice profiling, and the size and the diversity of our organization magnify all of them. The barriers we have experienced can be grouped into information technology and data issues, organization of care issues, and provider acceptance.

Our information systems offer both advantages and disadvantages. VA has maintained large amounts of clinical and administrative information in computerized databases for many decades and has been implementing a computerized medical record for the past 10 years. Consequently, large data sets are readily available. Until recently, however, much of these data were never considered very important and the quality of many data elements was problematic. We cannot stress enough the importance of automating and standardizing data collection and entry. In an effort to ensure the integrity of data elements, we developed *truth tables* against which extracted data were checked. For example, we crossed-checked the patient's age against the era of military service to ensure that it fell into mutually compatible ranges.

In addition to ensuring data integrity, we discovered how difficult it is to construct valid and reliable measures. Although we could easily define measures, ensuring that we reliably captured all data elements was a major undertaking. This required us to develop a number of business rules to ensure that data elements were collected and applied in a standardized fashion (e.g., what constitutes an active patient for the purposes of inclusion in the data analysis). Additionally, to construct population measures, we had to develop methods to pool utilization data from multiple sites.

In order to benchmark practice performance across our system, we also had to address a number of issues related to organization of care. Uniformity in the delineation of primary care provider responsibilities across all delivery sites was necessary in order to ensure that data elements and measures were valid, consistent, comparable, and reproducible. However, strict uniformity in our care delivery processes could only be achieved at a significant cost to the organization. Therefore, we sought to strike a balance between the optimal arrangements necessary to support a nationwide practice profiling initiative and the realistic need for local autonomy and flexibility. Ensuring that a single principal provider had continuity and responsibility for his or her panel of patients and the ability to control or significantly influence critical factors related to desired outcomes was a major undertaking. For example, primary care providers in most of our facilities had little control over utilization of subspecialty consultations, and this undermined the primary care provider's ability to direct care and maintain continuity. We knew that, without an ability to influence these processes and resources, responsible clinicians would most assuredly become disenfranchised and frustrated. We had to develop mechanisms and organizational models that supported our primary care clinicians in these new roles.

Although some clinicians have found practice management data interesting and useful, many have remained skeptical and have expressed significant concerns about the potential for inappropriate use of these data. In spite of our efforts to educate providers about practice management data, most clinicians had myriad unanswered questions. We significantly underestimated the level of anxiety and the degree to which clinicians would want detailed information about our methodologies and an opportunity for meaningful input. Implementation of practice profiling requires a significant investment in education to ensure comprehensive understanding of fundamental principles and data management strategies. Additionally, we believe educational material must accompany the practice profiles. This educational material should serve not only to inform clinicians about methodologies, but also to help them learn new ways to improve performance. We also found that clinicians became frustrated with the lack of robustness in our early data sets. Initially, we simply provided paper reports on a monthly basis to clinicians. Those whose performance was at either end of the spectrum had no ability to discover causes. This experience has reinforced our belief that we need data-mining tools and decomposable data sets if clinicians are to discover opportunities to improve performance.

Conclusions

The development of high-quality, provider-specific performance data has been an expensive and laborious undertaking. When all is said and done, we believe our efforts will improve the value of health care services we render to America's veterans. Defining responsibilities for clinical outcomes and resource utilization and managing accountability poses significant challenges and raises numerous philosophical and ethical issues. Furthermore, we recognize that physician performance is often just one component. As health care becomes more complex, outcomes will be based less on individual performance and more on the performance of teams and systems. We will effectively manage system performance only when we understand these processes and how the individual performance of various providers contributes to the outcomes we desire.

References

1. Kizer, K., and others. "The Veterans Healthcare System: Preparing for the Twenty-First Century." *Hospital and Health Services Administration* 42(3):283-98, Fall 1997.

2. Wennberg, J., and Gittelsohn, A. "Variations in Medical Care among Small Areas." *Scientific American* 246(4):120-34, April 1982.

3. Greco, P., and Eisenberg, J. "Changing Physicians' Practices." *New England Journal of Medicine* 329(17):171-3, Oct. 21, 1993.

4. Tompkins, C., and others. "Physician Profiling in Group Practices." *Journal of Ambulatory Care Management* 19(4):28-39, Oct. 1996.

5. Iezzoni, L., and others. "Comorbidities, Complications, and Coding Bias: Does the Number of Diagnosis Codes Matter in Predicting In-Hospital Mortality?" *JAMA* 267(16):2197-203, April 22-29, 1992.

6. McNeil, B., and others. "Current Issues in Profiling Quality of Care." *Inquiry* 29(3):298-307, Fall 1992.

7. Garnick, D., and others. "Focus on Quality: Profiling Physicians' Practice Patterns." *Journal of Ambulatory Care Management* 17(3):44-75, July 1994.

8. Shapiro, D., and others. "Containing Costs While Improving Quality of Care: The Role of Profiling and Practice Guidelines." *Annual Review of Public Health* 14:219-41, 1993.

9. Wray, N., and others. "Case-Mix Adjustment Using Administrative Databases: A Paradigm to Guide Future Research." *Medical Care Research Review* 54(3):326-56, Sept. 1997.

10. Berlowitz, D., and others. "Ambulatory Care Case-Mix Measures." *Journal of General Internal Medicine* 10(3):162-70, March 1995.

11. Averill, R., and others. *Design and Evaluation of a Prospective Payment System for Ambulatory Care.* Wallingford, Conn.: 3M Health Information Systems, 1990.

12. Weiner, J., and others. "Development and Application of a Population-Oriented Measure of Ambulatory Case-Mix." *Medical Care* 29(5):452-72, May 1991.

13. Duan, N., and others. "A Comparison of Alternative Models of the Demand for Medical Care." *Journal of Economics and Business* 35(2):115-26, April 1983.

James Tuchschmidt, MD, MBA, is Chief Executive Officer, Veterans Affairs Medical Center, Portland, Oregon. Carol M. Ashton, MD, MPH, is Director, Houston Center for Quality of Care and Utilization Studies, Veterans Affairs Medical Center, Houston, Texas.

CHAPTER 12

Profiling in an Academic Health Center

by Charles W. Mercer, MD, FACPE, John W. Lacey, MD,
and Francis Weisner, RN

*T*he University of Tennessee (UT) Medical Center in Knoxville, like most academic health centers, is in a transition from cottage industry to organized delivery of care. UT Medical Center is located in largely rural East Tennessee, which only recently has seen a significant switch in payer methods to capitation. The Medical Center itself is composed of a large tertiary care teaching hospital currently utilizing 450 beds and a Graduate School of Medicine with 170 residents and 11 programs split evenly between primary care and specialty training. The Medical Center also provides clinical experience for medical students and many other health professional students.

As managed care activity appeared and then accelerated in East Tennessee, the Medical Center recognized the need to change the scope of its organizational structure. As a result, University Health System (UHS) was created as an adjunct to the traditional organization. Among the services that UHS offers are an insurance program with 70,000 covered lives and a physician practice management organization currently providing services for 160 physicians, including most of the primary care physicians associated with the Medical Center. Through UHS, the Medical Center developed a partnership with another large provider organization to create an at-risk provider network (Tennessee Health Partnership), which manages 170,000 TennCare lives in a 16-county area of East Tennessee. In parallel, the physicians associated with the Medical Center were encouraged in their creation of a single signatory provider organization, University Physicians' Association (UPA). This organization is functionally an independent practice association (IPA) governed by the full-time and clinical faculty at the institution. In sum, these structural and organizational changes have created a "virtual" health care system. Throughout this structural change, there has been concomitant change in the breadth, depth, and source of physician performance analysis and reporting. What has remained a constant has been an institutional commitment to keep physician profiling within the domain of the profession.

Physician profiling actually began at the Medical Center in the late 1970s but the scope of the data was limited to the practitioner's own volume, outcomes, and hospital charges. During this era, physician profiles included only variations from care as identified during specific "audits" of a given diagnosis or procedure. In the mid-1980s, as a result of negotiation of a preferred provider organization (PPO) contract with Alcoa Aluminum Company of American (a large local employer), the Medical Center's medical staff agreed to begin utilizing a new data system. This data system, Mediqual's Medisgroups® (now known as Atlas®), offered a variety of comparisons of individual physician data to that in several national databases. In addition, the data were severity-adjusted for each patient, utilizing clinical characteristics independent of the diagnosis or procedural codes. Medical staff participation was encouraged by selecting a "champion" from each major clinical service to participate on a steering committee whose goals were to understand the data, plan and recommend its uses, and subsequently support its use and dissemination throughout the Medical Center. As the project evolved, this same group of physicians sponsored a semi-annual presentation of the Medical Center's outcomes and resource use to a team from Alcoa Aluminum Co.

The data continued to be used by each department's quality improvement committee to monitor trends at least quarterly at the department, service, and physician levels for all high-volume or high-risk diagnosis-related groups. In the early 1990s the data were very effective in the design of clinical pathways. Because participation in the pathway was voluntary at the Medical Center, having aggregate data on all cases provided a comparison of the differences in practice patterns among practitioners who were and were not using pathways. It was found that, by sharing this type of data, even the practice patterns of nonparticipating physicians began to change as much, if not as quickly, as those of their participating colleagues. Initial successes were found in the surgical practices, where procedures were done repeatedly by a small number of physicians. Pathways for medical patients were much more complex, with care provided by a larger number of physicians on multiple nursing units.

We believe that pathways have been successful when they offered a safety net for our practitioners, as well as a thoughtful, physician-directed plan to provide care in less time with less resource utilization and with better outcomes. The result of this type of physician profiling has been practice pattern change toward lower resource utilization attributable to routine, regularly scheduled, and unending use of data by members of our medical staff. We recognize in the changes observed that there were (and still are) external forces equally instrumental in lowering resource utilization. While once immune to competitive market pressures, the academic physicians found that they were increasingly asked to "pay their own way" and to compete for market share. These pressures have encouraged physicians to use feedback on performance to help establish a comparative or measurable edge, not only in private clinical activity but also in resident program clinical services.

The latest tool in providing physician feedback on performance has been Mediqual's Atlas Physician Profile®, comparing performance not only to that of peers, but also to performance of the previous year. A simple quadrant graph displays the ratios for length of stay and charges, both severity-adjusted for the practitioner's patient mix. This has received a mixed review by members of the medical staff, but it is resulting in modification of performance and behavior. One early result of this activity in the Internal Medicine Department has been the opportunity to dispel a myth that resident services were more costly in terms of total resource utilization than were private services. Physician evaluations by service group and hospitalwide have subsequently shown the opposite to be true.

An opportunity to broaden the scope of physician profiling to include more outpatient activity-previously available for our physicians only through outside or third-party payer reports that did not have UT Medical Center physician input or scrutiny for validity and therefore did not enjoy physician acceptance as a basis for behavior or practice change-has emanated from the Tennessee Health Partnership (THP). THP's board has 50 percent physician representation. Reporting to this board are several physician committees, some of which decide the format of all physician performance bonuses. THP has gleaned information from claims data from both inpatient and outpatient arenas. Information, including referral rates to specialists, pharmaceutical utilization, emergency department use by groups and individual physician patients, preventative service rates, and other data, is used to comparatively profile physicians and groups of physicians for purposes of rewarding bonuses. Comparative data are local, statewide, and national in scope. From this profiling, a bonus system has been established that fosters and rewards physicians' practice patterns identified as highly desirable by their colleagues. Primary care physicians direct the incentives for their colleagues and the specialty doctors decide their own incentives. Care is taken to ensure that less than 20 percent of the bonus is directed toward resource utilization, and that more is directed toward better screening for early detection, access, and patient satisfaction. Aappropriate use of mammography as well as immunization rates in children have increased as a result of this profiling with a feedback process.

In the THP network, peer review is not limited to physicians with academic appointments at the Medical Center. The THP network encompasses physicians scattered throughout a 16-county area. No differentiation is made between academic and nonacademic physicians in profiling. Rather, the focus is on standards of excellence in patient care and degree of target achievement agreed upon by physicians.

University Physician Association represents the physician arm of the virtual health system for the UT Medical Center. As a physician-owned and -managed for-profit corporation, UPA has signed global risk contacts for professional services. For these physicians—both academic and nonacademic alike—the need for physician performance analysis as a group and on an individual basis has taken on new stature. UPA has spent a significant portion of its resources in educating its members regarding their utilization patterns by DRG as compared not only to national data bases but also to local community hospitals by Major Disease Categories (MDCs). This information has become a powerful tool in this physician organization to effect change in practice patterns where needed. An example of this activity has been the use of specialist referral data from THP participation on a risk basis to change the pattern of referrals of low back pain patients to orthopedic surgeons by primary care physicians. With education and data, such referrals have diminished. Other referral patterns, such as routine evaluation of Attention-Deficit Hyperactivity Disorder (ADHD) children by neurology, have been modified as a result of profiling and reporting physician referral activity. This profiling is also being utilized to help shape future UPA membership invitations, especially to specialist physicians.

In summary, health care market changes, including risk contracting with its financial incentives and increasing competition for patient market share, have not spared the academic medical center, even in its rural East Tennessee manifestation. Our long-standing belief in the use of peer review as the proper methodology to monitor and achieve quality—and now value—has not changed. However, the scope and the sources of the data being utilized in this effort have broadened considerably, as have the methods of and opportunities for feedback to UT Medical Center physicians—and their acceptance of the feedback. Each part of our health care organization is using physician performance analysis to some degree to maintain high quality and lower resource utilization and to create marketplace value. These changes have occurred in a culture that insists that this activity be done by a peer group process. Whether the marketplace will allow this peer ownership to continue remains to be seen.

Charles W. Mercer, MD, FACPE, is Executive Vice Chancellor, University of Tennessee, Knoxville, Tennessee. Jack W. Lacey, MD, is Chief Medical Officer and Francis Weisner, RN is Director of Medical Management at the University of Tennessee Medical Center.

CHAPTER 13

The Pharmacy Benefits Manager Perspective

by George Fulop, MD, MSCM, Glen Stettin MD,
Wai Mo, Matt Donaldson

ccording to a 1994 study of Medicare data conducted by the federal General Accounting Office, drug misadventures (e.g., inappropriate prescribing, noncompliance, and misuse) cost the U.S. government more than $20 billion annually and other payers countless billions more.[1] As a health care entity in a position to address this problem, pharmacy benefit managers (PBMs) have a significant opportunity to improve the prescribing practices of physicians, reduce health care costs, and improve patients' lives. The largest PBMs are uniquely positioned to profile the prescribing practices of physicians across the United States to improve the quality of care, influence appropriate use of pharmaceuticals, and reduce costs. A handful of the largest PBMs administer benefits for 139 million of the 186 million Americans with coverage for prescription drugs.[2]

Further, each of these PBMs processes prescriptions written by virtually all prescribers in the United States. These large PBMs also process prescriptions for multiple large payers and may achieve physician practice penetration rates of 10 to 50 percent, depending on the geographic area involved. Through computerized networks of retail pharmacies and mail service pharmacies, large PBMs can be expert, data-driven managers of pharmacy care. Whereas proprietary retail chains are limited to a purview of data among their affiliated pharmacies, a PBM is able to monitor dispensing across multiple retail chains as well as independent and mail service pharmacies. Therefore, a PBM is better positioned to monitor and support optimal prescribing.

The capability of PBMs to monitor and manage aggregate medication usage—and collect data on patient outcomes—enables them to offer strategies, information, and analysis related to the marketplace's interest in improving outcomes of chronic disease states through health management programs. At a minimum, the PBM captures retail and mail prescription transaction data, including any dispensing activity involving use of the patient's prescription plan card at any of more than 55,000 retail pharmacies nationwide, and aggregates usage reports to support better management of the sponsor's prescription benefit. At their best, PBMs provide analysis and intervention capabilities needed to make prescriber profiling successful. With information collected from network databases, PBM physician profiling programs can provide both population and point-of-service accounts of clinicians' prescribing patterns in clinical and economic terms.

An effective profiling system needs to meet a number of key criteria. It must: be operationally compatible with point-of-service activity, demonstrate adherence to evidence-based guidelines, be focused above all else on quality of care, and address cost-effectiveness in the context of meeting these care objectives. Once these criteria have been met, the method of presenting information to physicians becomes key to supporting a successful profiling system. Profiling communications to physicians should be simple, brief, and flexible, enabling dissemination of information either face-to-face or via mail or fax, thereby accommodating the demanding workflow of the clinician and avoiding disruption of point-of-service dispensing of prescriptions.

Further, cost and utilization data need to be presented in comparison with regional and/or specialty-specific peer data. Profiles display an encapsulated comparison of the individual provider's prescribing practices to a benchmark or to credible clinical targets derived from well-accepted guidelines that make a clear differentiation between providers adhering to best practice guidelines and outliers.

Finally, profiles need to be actionable, covering a wide mix of prescribing situations while highlighting prescribing areas or categories that involve particularly large deviations from guidelines or plan specifications. Profiling communications that meet these guidelines will help provide the physician with a clear understanding of the opportunities for changes in prescribing and with a reliable tool for making patient care decisions.

This chapter will describe an example of physician prescribing profiles and discuss the opportunities for using PBMs to improve care and manage costs.

PBM Use of Physician Profiling

The capability of PBMs to manage prescription benefit systems through the use of formularies and drug utilization review evolved to include physician profiling. These capabilities were developed to meet the service needs of employers, unions, managed care organizations, and government health plans for improved and more affordable pharmaceutical care. Payers have demonstrated a mounting interest in vigorous and creative strategies to stabilize costs in a era of annual double-digit increases in prescription expenditures. Increasingly, payers are confronting a dilemma: either implement strategies to streamline benefits and promote efficiencies in prescription costs or face the prospect of eliminating coverage for their members entirely. Over the past several years, payers have employed transaction-based drug utilization review (DUR) interventions through their PBMs to help meet their quality and cost objectives. At the pharmacy, the PBM's claims processing system is used to evaluate in real time the incoming prescription claim against the patients' utilization history and the payer's administrative and clinical rules for managing the benefit. This evaluation of the medication request's appropriateness and safety can be done either concurrently, while the patient is at the pharmacy counter, or retrospectively, after dispensing.

Transaction-based strategies employed by payers through PBMs include retrospective drug utilization reviews. In retrospective DUR, physicians are sent letters, after the prescribing event, requesting that they evaluate the appropriateness of prescriptions in light of available data and change therapies as appropriate. Retrospective DUR is reasonably effective at changing prescriptions for individual patients—in up to 50 percent of cases in which a physician responds to the DUR letter, the physician agrees that a change in therapy is appropriate.[3] However, a more robust intervention is needed to address common overutilization issues. Another transaction-based strategy is prior authorization, which occurs at the time the patient seeks to have the prescription filled and requires administrative approval prior to dispensing.

Prescriber Summary Reports

A PBM, such as Merck-Medco, may develop a physician prescriber profiling report system that leverages the strengths of its transaction-based capabilities. These reports are developed on the basis of the information from our physician profiling system. Plan-specific clinical and economic rules based on a combination of best practice guidelines and payer medication benefit design are applied at the prescriber level. Over time, patterns emerge from the data about a physician's prescribing behavior. These patterns are communicated to physicians through individual reports that provide a quick reference guide that the physician can use to compare his or her practice to the plan's clinical care and cost objectives. For the physician who often has no idea as to whether or not an individual patient fills or refills a prescription, the aggregate data across the practice is often quite enlightening. Physicians who are involved in capitated or other risk-sharing plans or who are becoming part of physician practice management (PPM) firms may find the profile information useful in allocating resources.

Measures commonly used in the prescriber profile reports include number of patients; number of prescriptions; number of prescriptions per patient; prescriptions per member per month; ingredient cost (the primary substance in a prescription compound); ingredient cost per prescription; ingredient cost per member per month; percentage of generic prescriptions; percentage of single-source prescriptions; percentage of multi-source prescriptions; percentage of formulary compliance; percentage of prescriptions dispensed as written (DAW); key product usage (e.g., ranitidine/Zantac®); and key formulary chapter usage (e.g., ulcer therapy: antisecretory agents such as H2 receptor antagonists, proton pump inhibitors, etc.). These measures help give the provider a basis for adjusting his or her prescribing practices as appropriate. These changes can be documented and monitored via subsequent reports.

Reports may also provide prescribers with key clinical measures, such as volume and percentage of antibiotics prescriptions compared to their peers, adherence to generic dispensing, formulary preference or medication guidelines, and potential overutilization in certain treatment categories.

Overcoming the Pejoratives of "Report Cards"
Not surprisingly, many physicians dislike the pejorative term "Report Card." PBMs attempt to navigate a fine line between, on the one hand, providing the physician with useful information that supports enhanced and more affordable pharmacy care and, on the other hand, causing a negative reaction by physicians who may conclude that these prescribing guidelines represent dictates that usurp the physician's authority to make patient care decisions. Rather than usurping the physician's power, profiling reports and other communications can enhance the physician-patient relationship by offering pertinent, clinical, patient-focused information that optimizes prescribing within a practice and offers the added advantage of calling key information to the attention of the prescriber that he or she can use to enhance care of the patient at the point-of-service. In the end, the treating physician determines the appropriateness of care for an individual patient.

Many of today's practitioners clearly would benefit from such tools. The $20 billion in annual nationwide costs associated with inappropriate prescription use, as evidenced by Medicare data, is due not only to noncompliance but also to errors in prescribing.[2] Practitioners also face mounting cost pressures based either on the financial pressures of plan designs or on the economic structure of their own practices—e.g., their ability to manage capitation and at-risk contracts. Still, although the need is well-documented, physician profiling is only beginning to be established as an accepted, effective tool in the management of health care resources.

Reports to date on the outcomes of physician profiling initiatives describe minimal to modest impact on care and costs. Balas and colleagues conducted a meta-analysis of 12 randomized, controlled clinical trials involving 553 profiled physicians.[4] They concluded that profiling resulted in an improvement in clinical practice of 9 percent, a figure they considered "statistically significant, but showing minimal effect on utilization." However, the meta-analysis included only four studies of prescribing behavior interventions in slightly more than 200 physicians. Physician profiling efforts by PBMs have received minimal study to date.

Some of the acknowledged physician resistance to these tools stems from profiling devices that largely emphasize cost rather than care. In refining a profiling system, PBMs are striving to make clinical information the centerpiece of performance reports to the physician.

Clinical Case Studies

The PBM case study profiling process began with the development of a comprehensive set of clinical rules and prescribing guidelines designed for effective prescription management. For rules developed internally, independent Medical Advisory Boards and/or Pharmacy and Therapeutics Committees, each consisting of nationally recognized expert clinicians and academicians, reviewed and approved the profile's clinical content.

Provider Prescribing Reports are typically sent via mail with a cover letter, and are often customized with a managed care organization's or Blue Cross Blue Shield plan's logo and message. By customizing communications with the client's brand name, a PBM can take advantage of the direct relationship that the organization already has established with the physician. With so many communications delivered to physicians each day, clinicians often react to messages based on the relationship they have with the party delivering them. However, intervention by mail alone is not adequate. The profiles may also be hand-delivered by health plan staff or by regional medical directors or pharmacists. These PBM-employed physicians and pharmacists can meet with physician groups or individuals to explain the profiles and to educate physicians on the best practice guidelines.

The Provider Prescribing Report was designed on the basis of input from focus groups of practicing physicians in which they expressed what they wanted to see in these communications. First, they wanted a report that was short, simple, and easy to comprehend. Voluminous and complicated reports would not be read. Second, the report must be relevant, meaning that the report reflects the physician's behavior, that peer groups used for any comparisons are appropriate for the prescriber being profiled, and that any guidelines or performance

FIGURE 1

Provider**Prescribing**Report

[MMMC or Plan Logo]

John Q. Sample, M.D.
999 Main Street
Anytown, NJ 12345

Specialty: Family Practice
Period From: 07/01/97 to 12/31/97
[Plan Name: XYZ Health Plan]

Generic Prescribing

Step 1 **Please evaluate:** *Are there opportunities for you to increase the prescribing of generic equivalents?*

Step 2 **Please consider the following statistics based on our records from the last 6 months:**

Total number of prescriptions with generic equivalents: 167

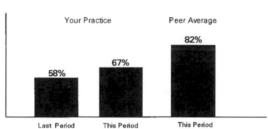

% of prescriptions with generic equivalents dispensed as generic

Step 3 **Please review these specific example**

Your Top Brand Medications by Savings Opportunity

Brand Products	Generic Alternatives	Number of Patients	Estimated Savings Opportunity	Savings %
Tagamet	cimetidine	15	$ 3,495.00	68%
Tenormin	atenolol	21	2,154.00	49%
Valium	diazepam	12	1,078.00	71%
Lasix	furosemide	9	678.00	62%
Motrin	ibuprofen	5	429.00	51%
Total estimated savings opportunity			$ 7,834.00	
Estimated PMPM savings opportunity			$ 21.06	

Next Steps

Please fill out the Response Form if you would like to:
✓ request a list of patients prescribed brand medications for evaluation
✓ provide comments on generic prescribing

Version A1.1   [Merck-Medco Managed Care, L.L.C. is a subsidary of Merck & Co., Inc.]

targets cited are ones with which the reasonable prescriber would agree. Irrelevant reports would not be read. Finally, the reports must be actionable, meaning that physicians wanted to be profiled on issues that were likely to present again, linked to specific prescribing benchmarks, and the profile must facilitate improvement in the physician's performance, if the provider agrees change is warranted.

The Provider Prescribing Report consists of a one-page summary of the physician's overall prescribing and supplementary pages devoted to specific therapeutic issues. The report is intended for quarterly distribution. The Provider Prescribing Report is modular, meaning that MMMC or the plan can choose which, if any, of the supplementary report pages to include. The summary page (figure 1, page 194) provides summary statistics, including per member per month prescription costs with prior period and peer comparisons. The supplementary pages provide more specific data and comparisons related to specific therapeutic issues, such as generic prescribing (figure 2, page 196). A particular therapeutic issue may involve both quality and cost issues in a single supplementary page. For example, if antidepressants were to be profiled, we may highlight an issue regarding potential underutilization (too short a duration of therapy) with an issue regarding potential overutilization (too long a duration of therapy).

A question or questions regarding prescribing behavior leads off the report. Second, the report summarizes the physician's prescribing practice and provides information on prescribing by peers for the therapeutic area identified. The third step of our report may contain a written description of the practice standard. Finally, the physician can 1) request additional details concerning patients included in the profile to facilitate possible changes in therapy, 2) request references regarding the prescribing standards, and 3) provide feedback on the report itself. Experience to date has found this approach to be much appreciated by physicians who have received the Provider Prescribing Report, with more than 9 out of 10 requesting that a new report be issued for the quarter following the initial delivery.[5]

To accommodate payer and physician needs, a PBM may also present aggregated prescriber activities of all plan physicians, e.g., a prescriber summary report that allows the plan's medical and pharmacy directors to monitor and support prescribing activities of affiliated physicians.

Discussion

Prior to the evolution in profiling technology spawned by PBMs, the typical primary care provider might treat 1,500 to 2,000 patients without a definitive, readily ascertainable picture of his or her overall prescribing performance. Even in the case of an individual physician interested in "self-auditing" his or

FIGURE 2

Provider**Prescribing**Report

[MMMC or Plan Logo]

John Q. Sample, M.D.
999 Main Street
Anytown, NJ 12345

Specialty: Family Practice
Period From: 07/01/97 to 12/31/97
[Plan Name: XYZ Health Plan]

Practice Summary

	Your Practice	Peer Average
Utilizing Member Profile:		
(Patients who filled one or more prescriptions during this report period)		
Number of utilizing members	83	104
Average age	53	59
Gender - % Female	55%	51%
% Male	45%	49%

Prescribing Summary:		
Total cost of prescriptions	$ 12,519	$ 13,141
Total number of prescriptions	227	208
Average number of distinct medications per utilizing member	3	2

Prescription Cost Statistics:		
Average cost per 30-days of therapy	$ 28.53	$ 25.30
Brand prescriptions	$ 33.04	$ 28.74
Generic prescriptions	$ 10.92	$ 10.13

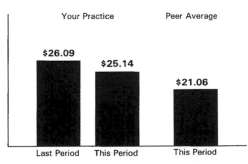

Cost per utilizing member per month

	Your Practice		Peer Average
	$26.09	$25.14	$21.06
	Last Period	This Period	This Period

Version A1.1   [Merck-Medco Managed Care is a subsidiary of Merck & Co., Inc.]

her practice's prescribing trends, the amount of time, organizational effort, and energy required to generate even the most rudimentary prescribing activity report would make the task impractical. Likewise, in the case of examining care for specific patients, physicians would not-without the benefit of PBM technology-gain a glimpse of what medications their patients may have had prescribed by other physicians for other treatment conditions and would have no information whatsoever on prescribing patterns among their colleagues.

PBMs are helping to advance the practice of physician profiling to a more refined, customized, and comprehensive tool for evaluating how physicians prescribe and to establish a foundation for peer comparison and improvement. The capability of PBMs in accumulating and sorting large amounts of data for the purpose of differentiating and evaluating prescribing patterns—on both a per physician and a per patient basis—was not routinely achievable in the past. Standardized electronic medical records now make it possible both to gain an in-depth look at a specific physician's prescribing patterns and to develop profiles based on a more universal practice perspective that takes into account hundreds of thousands and potentially millions of patient transactions involving prescribers facing similar treatment situations. Databases also make it possible to incorporate prescribing guidelines established by leading medical organizations to gain a glimpse of how their prescribing compares to widespread practice standards as documented by point-of-care data.

PBM advances in physician profiling should also provide a helpful tool for health plans seeking to document improvements in the quality of care within their practices, especially for the purpose of preparing HEDIS® data or to demonstrate progress in treating certain disease conditions in building a case for NCQA accreditation.[6] It's possible through the use of this tool not only to provide documentation of improved adherence to prescribing standards among affiliated plan physicians but also to generate reports and analyses documenting reductions in hospitalization rates and emergency department visits. For example, lowering the incidence and severity of adverse drug reactions increases medication adherence and consequently reduces medical resource use.

The future implications of employing such tools throughout medical practice will yield far more than a greater understanding of which physicians are adhering to best practice prescribing guidelines. The ability of this technology to link and interrelate drug and medical utilization data will enable physicians to go beyond making more informed prescribing choices to obtaining a comprehensive, outcomes-based practice tool that looks at and evaluates pharmacy care in the context of a full range of treatment options. Such technology is clearly useful not just in identifying the right drug to treat the right condition in the right patient, but also in comparing and contrasting a wide variety of treatment strategies using outcomes studies conducted among patients with similar chronic disease conditions. Through this technology, it might be possible not only to compare aggregate results of pharmacy care versus surgery, but also to evaluate the impact of patient and physician education programs, as well as preventive health care strategies such as diet and exercise, on overall medical utilization rates and patient outcomes.

The utility of PBM technology can only be enhanced and made more valuable as information shared via the convenience of the Internet accelerates the accumulation of knowledge and the pace of learning among both physicians and patients about appropriate use of pharmacy care in the treatment of specific disease conditions. In the future, physicians may increasingly find themselves logging onto specialized medical association and clinical practice Web sites to keep themselves apprised of the latest pharmacy-based outcomes studies, especially in evaluating the effectiveness of new or controversial prescription alternatives. This technology also holds the promise of eventually streamlining the physician profiling process to the point that some of the tutorial information that prescribers now receive in periodic summary profiling reports may be updated and incorporated into individual patient electronic medical records for access and use by the physician the next time that patient shows up for treatment.

Conclusion

Most physicians would probably agree with the essential goals of profiling: to reduce inappropriate and wasteful variation in prescription practice and to improve the quality of patient care. However, some physicians have had negative experiences with profiling in the past, and PBMs developing profiling capabilities must contend with these negative impressions in the physician community. The challenge is to appeal to the physician's sense of patient-centric, best-practice medicine and resource-efficient economics. Information provided by PBM profiling reports will not only enable physicians to be better caregivers on a one-to-one patient level but will also help them understand aggregate disease trends within their entire patient base. The economics of appropriate prescribing is presented in the context of best practice guidelines. To the extent that physician profile reports are based on clinically and educationally sound prescribing fundamentals, buttressed by solid economics, physicians will be more receptive to the message. When well-executed physician profiling programs support physician decision making and create costs savings by managing utilization, they are important contributors to effective health care.

References

1. *Prescription Drugs and the Elderly.* Washington, D.C.: United States General Accounting Office, Health, Education, and Human Services Divisions-95-152, 1995.

2. *Pharmacy Benefit Management.* Palo Alto, Calif.: Health Strategies Group, Inc., April 1998, Section IV, p. 6

3. From Merck-Medco Managed Care data files.

4. Balas, E., and others. "Effect of Physician Profiling on Utilization. Meta-Analysis of Randomized Clinical Trials." *Journal of General Internal Medicine* 11(10):584-90, Oct. 1996

5. From Merck-Medco Managed Care data files.

6. Draft HEDIS® 1999 Standards. Washington, D.C.: National Committee for Quality Assurance, 1998. Draft developed under auspices of the Committee on Performance Measures for public comment, April 15-May 29, 1998.

George Fulop, MD, MS, is Senior Director of Medical Policy and Programs; Glen Stettin, MD, is Vice President of Utilization Management; Wai Mo, is Senior Director of Audience/Channel Development; and Matt Donaldson, is Vice President of Audience/Channel Development, Merck-Medco Managed Care, L.L.C., Franklin Lakes, N.J.

INDEX

A

academic health center, 185
accounting problems, 117
accreditation, 90
ACG, 44
Acute physiological and chronic health evaluations, 44,75,109,110
ADG, 44
Agency for Health Care Policy and Research (AHCPR), 9
aggregation problem, 112
all patient refined diagnosis-related groups, 44
All Patient Refined DRGs, 75
all-payer diagnosis-related groups, 44
ambulatory care groups, 44, 180
ambulatory diagnostic groups, 44, 110
ambulatory patient groups, 75,180
ambulatory visit groups, 75
American College of Physicians, 27
American Health Information Management Association, 92
American Medical Accreditation Program, 27
American Medical Association, 26,27
American Medical Association, 27
Anderson Area Medical Center, 135
APACHE, 44,75,109,110
Atlas Physician Profile, 187
autonomy, 5

B

benchmarking, 46
Best Doctors, 56

C

captured audience syndrome, 103

care environment, 123
case mix, 30,41,74,179
Center for Research in Ambulatory Health Care Administration, 76
claims data, 24,117
clinical guidelines, 9,156
coding, 38,120
Codman, Ernest, 18
collective bargaining, 5
comorbidity, 120
Computerized Severity Index, 75,109,11110
confidentiality, 89
consent, 90
Consumers for Quality Care, 95
continuous quality improvement (CQI), 45,64,75,10,150
control charts, 45
cost data, 39
credentialing, 25,92,155,158

D

dashboard indictor reports, 71
data edits, 38
data integration, 104
Department of Veterans Affairs, 169
diagnosis-related groups, 27,44,103,109,188
diagnostic clusters, 75
diagnostic cost groups, 45
diagnostic episode Cluster, 109, 119
disaggregation problem, 112
discovery, 57
disease interactions, 120
disease management, 10
disease staging methods, 44,75
drug utilization reviews, 191
drugs, 189
Duke University, 108

E

economic credentialing, 94
economic profiling, 150
economies of scale, 104
education, 135
electronic medical record, 150,159
employed physician, 4

episode treatment group, 27,45,109, 119
episode treatment groups, 27
episodes of care, 118,120
evidence-based medicine, 63,76

F

feedback, 135,164,172
fraud and abuse, 54

G

General Accounting Office, 189
Glasgow Coma Scale, 109
group practice, 4,6,149,161

H

Harvard Community Health Plan, 161
Harvard Pilgrim Health Care, 161
Health Care Financing Administration, 18,30
Health Care Quality Improvement Act of 1986, 93, 97
Health Insurance Experiment, 108
Health Insurance Portability and Accountability Act of 1996, 91
Health Outcomes Institute, 108
Health Plan Employer Data and Information Set, 9,47,73
Health Quality Choice Coalition, 49
Health Risk Adjustment Study, 45
Healthnet vs. Weiss Research Inc., 96
HEDIS, 9,47,73,103

I

IBNR, 40
IM System, 73
incurred but not reported, 40
Informatics, 101
information systems, 182
institutional practice, 4
Internet Directories, The , 56
Internet, 53,91

J

Joint Commission on Accreditation of Healthcare Organizations, 73,90

L

libel, 95

M

Maine Medical Malpractice Demonstration Project, 87
major disease categories, 188
malpractice, 5,86
managed care, 8,24,47,88,161
Massachusetts profiling, 53
Medicaid study, 57
medical complications, 115
Medical Group Management Association, 27,57
Medical Outcomes Study, 108
Medicare + Choice, 45
Medicare, 7,18,30
medications, 189
MedisGroups, 44,75,110,186
merger, 161
misuse of profiling, 57
Mortality Probability Models, 109
mortality rates, 19,41
multiple-environment model, 124
N
National Claims History File, 31
National Committee for Quality Assurance, 27,73,90
negligence, 88
New Jersey DRGs, 109
norm, 20

O

Organ-System Failure Model, 109
ORYX, 73
outcome measures, 22,73
outcomes, 21
outliers, 38,88

P

pathways, 186
patient classification, 180
patient management categories, 44
patient satisfaction, 157
peer review organizations (PROs), 7
peer review, 93
Pennsylvania Corporate Hospital Rating Project, 49
per member per month, 39

performance improvement, 52
pharmacy benefits manager, 189
pharmacy, 189
physician impatient resource score, 70
Physician Organization Certification Program, 27
Physician Payment Review Commission, 19
physician selection, 53,153
physician unions, 5
physiology-based severity adjustment, 109
Pilgrim Health Care, 161
plan-do-study-act cycle, 76
PMC, 44
PMPM, 39
population at risk, 48
practice guidelines, 9,156
practice patterns, 18,79,135,170
practice style factor, 30
practice variation, 19,41,169
practiced-based norm, 20
prescribing practices, 189
primary care physician, 11,40,49,107
principal inpatient procedure-diagnostic cost groups, 45
principal-care physician, 26
process measures, 22
professional autonomy, 5
professional standards review organizations (PSROs), 7
professional standards, 6
profile elements, 39
profiling rate, 20
prospective payment system, 7
provider performance assessment, 20
provider prescribing report, 193

Q

quality assurance, 7,150
Quality Compass, 46,47,73
quality improvement, 20,173
quality measures, 22

R

RAND Corporation, 108
rates, 40
ratios, 40

recredentialing, 155
relative value units, 57,103
reliability, 44,170
report cards, 47,136,157,192
resource utilization, 26
resource-based severity adjustment, 109
Rhode Island profiling, 56
Rickabaugh case, 95
risk adjustment, 25,37,41,75,118,179
risk appraisals, 87
risk vs. severity, 125
risk, 125
Robert Wood Johnson Foundation, 57

S

sampling error, 39
severity adjustment, 108
severity of illness, 44,74,118,171
severity, 125
sharing profiles, 23
Simplified Acute Physiology Score, 109
single-environment model, 124
small numbers, 74
Society of Actuaries, 45
specialty care practice, 12
Standardized Hospitalization Ratios, 151
Standardized Mortality Ratios, 151
Standardized Transplantation Ratios, 151
standards setting, 6
Starr, Paul, 3
statistical process measures, 45

T

Tennessee Health Partnership, 187
timeliness, 171
total quality management, 45
trade libel, 95
treatment algorithms, 126

U

United Healthcare, 52
University of Pittsburgh study, 57
University of Tennessee, 185

utilization data, 39
Utilization Review and Accreditation Commission, 90
utilization review, 7,20
utilization, 26

V

validity edits, 38
validity, 170
validity, 43

W

Watson Clinic, 149